"Knowledge is power and MonkeyBrain places power directly in the hands of its readers, delivering a clear understanding between the brain, body, and spirit connections. It provides a wealth of information as well as a practical plan of action for growth and development in all areas. The Joyefit Fusion provides the means for sustainable positive change."

~ Gina Jo Kraus, CCP Personal Empowerment life Coach

"MonkeyBrain is the bible for the brain and a must read for every practitioner! It merges science, psychology, medicine and inspires a transformation of consciousness"

~ Jaclyn Shedded, MSN, FNP-C, Nurse Practitioner

"MonkeyBrain is like having a private lifestyle fitness coach at your disposal. For many years Johnny worked with me and my business in the franchise health club industry, developing and implementing wellness and athletic programs. Many years later his vision and passion to help others remains the same. MonkeyBrain shares his unique style of coaching ensuring a successful balance. Johnny explains how brain chemicals impact our emotions and physical health and provides ways to improve and maintain a healthy balance. In addition, MonkeyBrain provides a pathway to improve the physical body while helping to create spiritual awareness and development. The twenty-one day challenge is a great personal growth guide for any fitness professional or others trying to improve mentally, physically, or spiritually."

~ Anna Paula Azirovic, Fitness and Wellness Professional

# MonkeyBrain

*Create Emotional Balance, Physical
Health, and Spiritual Awareness*

*Brain – Body – Spirit
The Practical Approach*

JOHNNY OYE

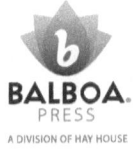

BALBOA.
PRESS
A DIVISION OF HAY HOUSE

Balboa Press books may be ordered through booksellers or by contacting:

Balboa Press
A Division of Hay House
1663 Liberty Drive
Bloomington, IN 47403
www.balboapress.com
1 (877) 407-4847

Printed in the United States of America.

ISBN: 978-1-4525-1948-7 (sc)
ISBN: 978-1-4525-1950-0 (hc)
ISBN: 978-1-4525-1949-4 (e)

Library of Congress Control Number: 2014913746

Balboa Press rev. date: 9/12/2014

# Contents

# Foreword

John Oye's first book is the culmination of his twenty years of experience as a personal trainer and lifestyle fitness coach. This experience led him to understand that we all react to imbalances and stress in much the same way. He wanted to know what ruled our moods, what makes us feel strong or weak. Why could we be all these things at different times in our lives? Better yet, how can we improve this balance and optimize our well-being? More importantly, how can we control our MonkeyBrain that always wants to create imbalance?

*MonkeyBrain* is an incredible journey of discovery that began when Oye started exploring the relationships between our brain, our body, and our spirit. By creating his Joyefit Fusion system, the author was able to map out a path to well-being between these systems. What he learned was the MonkeyBrain in all of us cannot be defeated; rather, it can only be patrolled, and that control comes with optimizing balance.

Oye knows that getting from here to there first means understanding what the MonkeyBrain is and how important it is to tame it.

Next, he takes us on a journey that tells us about the brain. Here, the author explains how the brain reacts chemically to the information coming in from the universe, both inside and outside our bodies. It is a wonderful reference section that is highly readable and informative. You'll find yourself reviewing it time and again.

Assessing and conditioning your physical body is the next great tutorial that will help balance your brain, body, and spirit. Here is a wealth of information that you will refer to often on your way to optimum health.

Finally, Oye gives us a great overview of our spirits and his surprising and convincing discussion on the importance of spiritual practices to optimize health.

The book, *MonkeyBrain*, connects all the dots here with brain (chemical), body (physical), and mind (spiritual) connections that will make sense. It includes worthy projects for improving your life.

Last but not least, the author has included his template for everyone to use. It is called the Joyefit Fusion, a twenty-one day challenge.

Here you will be able to systematically work on optimum balance and well-being by doing brain work, body work, and spirit work on a daily basis for twenty-one days! Have fun and enjoy the Fusion!

Patricia Smith
Content Editor
For many years Patricia Smith produced tech manuals for assembling complex systems for an Aerospace Company. Twenty years later, she became Municipal Clerk and Treasurer in Vermont where she prepared Annual Town Reports about the towns business and financial status. Fifteen years later, Smith was elected to the Vermont House of Representatives. Presently she restores old homes.

# Dedication

*MonkeyBrain* is dedicated to my friend, my mentor, and my fellow SOULdier of the light, Gina Jo Kraus. Her leadership in the area of mindful living has inspired so many of us to continue to spread the majik to everyone by following our inner compass. Her mission, using Got the Secret, serves to unite mankind on a global scale, emphasizing *oneness*.

Gina's patented symbolic inner compass is a powerful symbol, created as a means to recognize those who choose to think, speak, and act in the positive—those working with all their good from within, who are thereby changing our world.

Gina shows her commitment to helping others find their way by making those who have Got the Secret not such a secret through display of the Symbolic Inner Compass, thereby encouraging interaction and success! I am forever grateful to you for allowing me to brand my body with your symbol, reminding me to strive for positivity in all aspects of my life. The symbol can be found at www.gtscollection.com and is forever tattooed on my arm.

Thank you, Gina Jo!

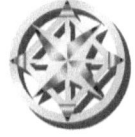

# Acknowledgments

First and foremost, I would like to thank my dear friend and editor, Patricia P. Smith. This book would not have been possible without her help and support. Thank you for believing in me and special thanks for your endless hours of helping me edit, and re-edit until we got it right. I will be forever grateful to you for inspiring and challenging me to share this vision. Thank you, Patty!

I am also very grateful to the countless authors, professors, and teachers who inspired me through their perspectives, insights, and knowledge. Thank you!

I would like to offer special thanks to those who literally changed my life with their teachings. Thank you Eckart Tolle, Dr. Wayne Dyer, Dr. C. J. Jung, Professor Sam Wang, Professor Peter Satterfield, Dr. Richard Restek, Dr. Deepak Chopra, and Jerry & Esther Hicks

I would also like to thank my family and friends for always being supportive and understanding.

Last, I would like to give a big thanks to all of my amazing clients who cared and supported me throughout this process. Thank you, all!

## Acknowledgments

# Preface

For over two decades, I have worked in the wellness industry as a certified trainer and lifestyle fitness coach, helping others improve their health and physiques. To this day, I continue to work one-on-one with clients on a daily basis.

*MonkeyBrain* is the result of many of years of research where I eventually discovered the connection between the brain, the body, and the spirit. This journey shares what I learned and also provides a plan of action. While helping my clients improve their physical health, I began to see and to understand that emotional well-being had a direct impact on physical and spiritual health. This also included social and cultural factors that are also often relevant to health, such as the environment, behavior, and stressful lifestyles.

To my surprise, stress was the biggest challenge to overall wellness for most, and MonkeyBrain is the term that I will use to describe the emotional reaction to stress.

MonkeyBrain is what happens when things aren't going your way, or for anything that upsets you and makes you feel powerless, angry, vindictive, or trapped. It is going a little crazy and a little out of control with your thoughts and actions. If left unchecked, your brain will bring other past examples of like behavior to the forefront in order to prove why you *deserve* to go out of control. And *bam*, your MonkeyBrain is now in charge. Sound familiar?

Many years ago, I began to notice undeniable patterns among my clients. Upon reflection, I also noticed these patterns in myself. What became apparent, time and time again, was that most of us tend to spiral into negative thinking when we are stressed. It almost seemed like an addiction, a worst-case scenario addiction. The stories that I heard, over and over, were mostly about bad news, drama, and disappointment. I heard much more of the negative stories than positive ones. Even when I did hear positive, uplifting stories, perhaps about a wedding or another joyous event, the story also included the drama.

What intrigued me most was that many of these stories were about past events that still carried a lot of negative emotion. Many of us seem to have this compulsion to relive old problems. If it wasn't old problems, it was pessimism or fear of the future. I include myself in this way of thinking as I often found myself wanting to share my sad story while listening to my client's bad day.

I also noticed that the content of our conversations changed as my clients began to exercise. The shift in brain chemistry, triggered by exercise, reduced their stress levels and allowed them to see things differently. It became clear to me that it was not so much about the original stress, but more about how we cope with that stress. I still wondered why we engaged in this stinking thinking in the first place. I began to call this way of thinking MonkeyBrain, and so I set off on a mission to find the MonkeyBrain fix.

My background in physiology did not prepare me for these challenges, and so I started to study the brain, learning as much about brain functions as possible. I wanted to know why we all tend to think negative thoughts more often than positive ones. My question was, why do we have this compulsion to relive these bad experiences over and over in our heads, and also share these memories with others?

What I learned was not only surprising but life-changing. This insight inspired me to share what I learned to help others understand why we do this and, more important, how to control or at least shrink the MonkeyBrain outbreaks!

Quickly, I discovered that improving our physical bodies was not enough. Overall wellness is much more complicated. A healthy physical body was only part of the puzzle. I realized that we were emotional and spiritual beings, I knew these factors had to be addressed. Eagerly, I looked at the latest research in psychology, neuroscience, and brain chemistry. I also studied the latest research on the connection between spritualty, health, and disease. Most of the research focused on three factors: What makes us sick? What makes us well? And what can we do to make it better?

I now began to suspect that imbalances of the brain, body, and spirit have a negative and dramatic affect on our overall health. I wanted to know what we can do to improve each while maintaining overall balance. This is where my journey began. I slowly discovered the missing pieces to that puzzle called life.

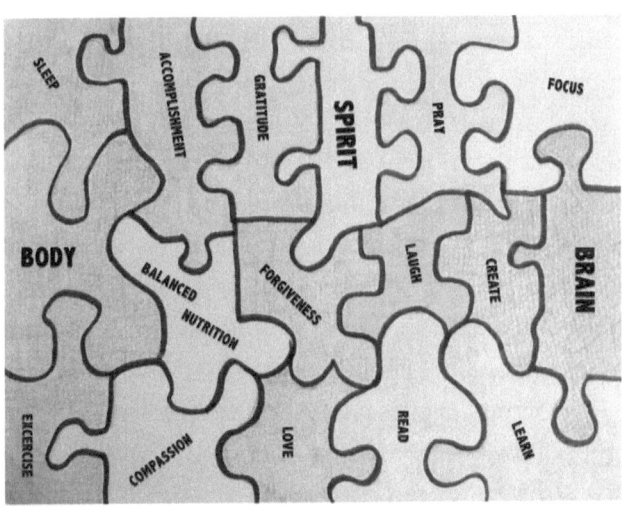

## The Puzzle of Life

The puzzle helped me recognize what I needed to add to my life in order to create emotional balance. Once I filled in the blanks of this puzzle, I then slowly began to develop a program to improve The overall balance and well-being of the entire human system. The Joyefit Fusion workout was born.

The intent of MonkeyBrain is to first help you understand how the brain works and how the body reacts. Understanding how the brain works can help us enhance positive experiences and reduce the negative ones. Personal growth requires a plan and participation. Each part will provide you with the necessary framework to help you establish a structured plan of action for growth and change in all areas.

We will explore the *brain, body, and spirit connection,* as well as review the functions and chemicals of the brain. Also we will touch on the role of the subconscious and unconscious. In addition, we will define the brain and the mind, highlighting their differences and unique yet integrated roles and controls.

To understand the concept of different roles for the brain and for the mind is to think of the mind as the driver of the vehicle and the brain as the engine. Once you think about it, you can get a glimmer of the role of the driver making sure the engine and the body are well taken care of with the proper maintenance. Just like a finely-tuned automobile engine needs maintenance—oils, gas, and fluids—the human engine (the brain) needs maintenance as well, with proper movement, balanced nutrition, and sufficient sleep. The driver (the mind) can and should be a gentle, caring steward of the engine's well-being.

Part I of Monkey Brain will investigate the brain with an overview of systems and functions that affect our overall health. This overview includes topics such as brain chemistry, the stress response, emotions, behavior, and how memory works.

In addition, we will look at what I believe to be one of the main causes of disease: *stress!* Here we explore the cause and effects of stress and ways to *reduce it.* Then look at ways to improve brain function in areas of memory and the ability to focus and concentrate. Part II will address the physical body, including nutritional needs, and ways to *improve possible deficits.* Finally, Part III explores the connection between spirituality and our health.

## How to Use This Book

MonkeyBrain is broken down into three parts: brain (neuroscience/psychology), body (physiology), and spirit (energy/physics). This will help you understand the functions and processes of all three. At the end of each part, you can participate in testing and assessments that will determine where you are now. Once you have determined your strengths and weaknesses, you can move on to the conditioning programs. Each part will provide a plan of action, which will include tools, techniques, or exercises designed to improve that specific discipline.

At the end of Part III is a twenty-one day Joyefit Fusion challenge. This journal is provided so you can document your participation, progression, and results. The journal is a great tool to keep you on track and help structure your personalized program. It is designed for personal growth by improving the complete human system:

brain, body, and spirit. The goal is to move beyond wellness and create wholeness. So let's get started!

# Introduction

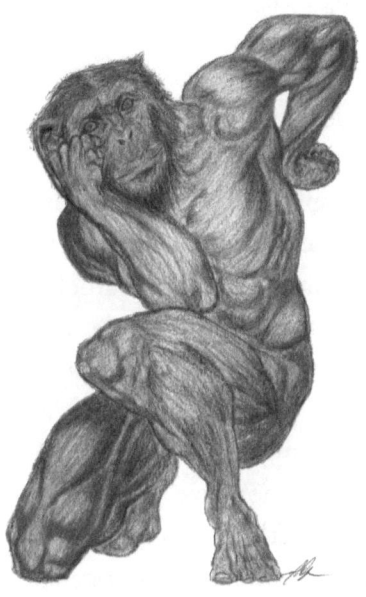

*The purpose of life is to live it, to taste experience*
*to the utmost, to reach out eagerly and without*
*fear for newer and richer experiences.*
*~ Eleanor Roosevelt*

For the last two decades, my life was focused on learning and teaching how the body worked, and ways to improve it. Throughout those years, while working in the fitness industry, I practiced countless fads that promised the best physical results. I tried just about every new workout that targeted physical fitness, from spinning to yoga and everything in between. I tried every fad diet, from high protein/low carb to low calorie/low fat. They all worked when the programs were followed as recommended. However, there were additional components to include; otherwise, the programs didn't work. Most of the diet plans recommended exercise, and most of the exercise programs recommended balanced nutrition. What resulted was that none of the programs really worked long-term without the other components.

Let's take the Atkins low carb/high fat diet into consideration. The recommended diet works to lose body fat very well but doesn't provide the necessary balance of nutrients to fuel the brain for optimum function. Eventually, it becomes difficult to maintain the diet because there is a sense of hunger that is difficult to pinpoint. The lack of carbohydrates is part of what creates the imbalance that leaves the brain hungry. Since the brain and the body require a certain amount of carbohydrates, this diet leaves you yearning for more. What I found was that most of these programs lacked balance. Those hunger pangs just didn't go away. I may not have been hungry for food or physical health, but I felt something was missing. How many times have you found yourself looking in the refrigerator for more food to eat even though you just had a full meal? We hunger for many things, including love, purpose, and accomplishment. In other words, conditioning and improving the physical body just so that we can look better is not enough. Nor is it enough to improve the intellect just to be smart. Also, developing the spirit without addressing the health of the brain and body is not enough. Working one without the others will create temporary results, at best. Well-being requires that we condition the whole. And what I mean by whole is mental and emotional balance, physical strength and health, and spiritual awareness. *MonkeyBrain* is designed to help create that balance.

My personal journey began at a young age with physical fitness, running, and weight training. Later, in my adult years, I added some mental conditioning (brain training), and finally, I went down the path of spiritual development. I didn't exclude organized religion or its teachings; rather, I began to look into the practices that I thought could lead me forward spiritually. Similar to the way I approached brain and body conditioning, I also began to experiment with many different techniques that were known as *spiritual work*, such as, meditation, yoga, and the practice of gratitude. In addition to practicing these disciplines, I also reviewed the latest research that looked at the health benefits of each. All of these had positive effects on brain chemistry, the cardiovascular system, and on the nervous system.

I found the spiritual work was very different than what I had been used to with physical and mental training. This work was more about slowing the brain's activity. I first tried yoga and noticed changes in my stress levels after a few weeks of practice. Now my questions were: Were these physical movements and balance poses causing changes to my brain and body? Were there psychological and biological changes happening as well? I decided to introduce more of these activities. First, I began a gratitude journal (which has become a daily practice). Next, I put some time into the practice of meditation. I tried different music, mantras, and breathing techniques, and yet I still could not shut my thoughts off. As a matter of fact, I had more thoughts. Instead of feeling relaxed after meditation, I felt annoyed.

One day, I tried something different. I did my physical workout in a specific order and ended the workout with meditation and writing in my gratitude journal. What I realized was the sequence in which I did the exercises made a big difference. I actually felt the difference. My body felt strong yet relaxed. This is when I started experimenting with combining different disciplines into one workout and realized that we can influence the chemical balance of our brain and body with specific movements and behavior. After I spent some time practicing countless combinations of disciplines, what resulted was a fusion workout that conditions the whole: brain, body, and the spirit. More details on the fusion in Part II and III, but for now, let's get back to the brain. In addition to the changes that I was feeling, I was most intrigued by the fact that I looked at things differently. My focus was more on the solutions to the problems instead of allowing my brain to think about the problem. I wanted to know specifically what I was doing that was creating these changes. At this point, I began to evaluate my activity and behavior, and used the process of elimination to identify how each made me feel, individually and collectively.

My question now was: Were the changes I was experiencing because of the spiritual work I was practicing or was there more to this? Was the link between physical and mental work symbiotically creating a new and better wellness? These questions will be answered throughout *MonkeyBrain*. The processes and the techniques I found most effective will be provided in later chapters. What I will be sharing with you is many years of learning, practicing, and discovering how the brain works and how the body reacts or responds. In addition, we will review the latest research that shows the power of positive thinking, prayer, meditation, and gratitude on our overall health.

First, I want to help you understand how the brain works. Once you understand this overview, we will look at the physical body and how to condition it. Finally, we will talk about the spirit in all of us. My original intent was to teach others how to use physical fitness and proper nutrition to improve their health and physiques.

During the process and research, I discovered much more than I had anticipated. What I learned was that all of our emotions and behavior are driven by our body's chemicals and hormones.

Physical fitness and balanced nutrition were only two parts of the puzzle.

Surprisingly, there were many non-physical activities that stimulate positive, rewarding chemicals that I was not aware of. These activities included things such as compassion, acts of service, and forgiveness. Brain chemicals determine how we feel: good, bad, or indifferent. Every thought, action, reaction, or response that we have has a direct effect on our brain/body balance. After reviewing the latest research on the health benefits of these non-physical activities, I felt compelled to share this data as well. The more I learned about and practiced this spiritual work, the more *MonkeyBrain* evolved.

At this point, I focused on what we could do that would influence our health in a positive manner. I wanted to discover ways to improve our strength and our drive to succeed in all things. I also wondered what stopped us from succeeding and why we continued down false paths that resulted in the failure to obtain our goals. I was looking for those answers that were not so obvious.

I eventually realized we are who we are because of biological, psychological, social, and cultural factors. All of these things influence our beliefs, our habits, and our personalities. Fortunately, because of *brain plasticity* (the ability to change and re-map brain patterns), most of this can be changed at any time during our lifetime. Most of what we feel is determined by the chemical balance of our brain, and those chemicals are known as neurotransmitters and hormones. Later on, we will review these chemicals, but first I would like to explain what triggered my interest. What I witnessed, time after time, was that most of us react emotionally to life's experiences instead of responding intuitively.

In other words, most of us react first and then think, instead of thinking first then responding. How many times have you said something that you wished you hadn't said? Always say it in your head before you say it out loud. The wrong words and tone can cut deeper than the sharpest knife.

We develop behavior based on patterns and connections in the brain. These patterns and connections become behavioral circuits. These circuits become conditioned reactions or responses to another person, place, or thing. For instance, social anxiety is a stress pattern that has been conditioned over time and has become a behavioral circuit. The fear of flying can be a conditioned pattern. This reactive behavior dictates our lives in a number of ways, such as our negative or positive reaction to others and our emotional stability or instability. It includes how we think and feel about ourselves. For example, feeling insecure or feeling superior can be a conditioned pattern. No one is born with an inferiority or superiority complex; it is conditioned over time. The conditioning begins at a very early age, but these patterns can last a lifetime. Another example would be an angry reaction to a person when they push your buttons. The slightest triggers can cause you to react before thinking. This emotionally charged behavior is what I call MonkeyBrain. Chapter 1 will explore the meaning in detail.

I could see that these unfettered reactions or responses will and do affect most people's health in negative ways. This made me take a deeper look into the latest research available. First, I looked at neuroscience, which gave me the latest information on how the brain works. Second, the study of physiology shows us how the body functions and ways to improve it. And finally, physics gave me insight on how everything begins with energy. This includes human energy. This is the energy that we excrete and others around us feel. Be aware of your energy, because that energy will affect every other person that you encounter.

When we study and learn the entire human system, we can see the bigger picture. Once I understood the entire system, I could see the connection between the brain, body, and spirit.

I was soon convinced that these three sciences were interdependent and connected. Together, they could also be known as the brain, body, and spirit connection, but we call it the Joyefit Fusion.

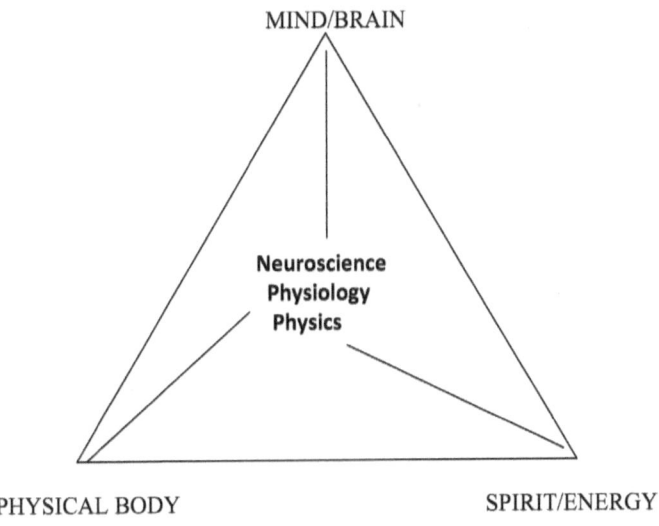

The interaction and the connection of these three determine our health as a whole. How we influence each determines the balance as a whole.

Now let's move on to Part I on the brain.

# PART I

# *The Brain*

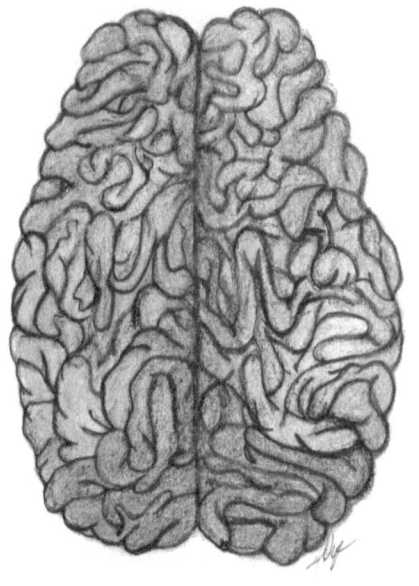

*The mind, not the brain, is the origin of consciousness. No mechanical explanation working from facts about the brain suffices.*
*~ Deepak Chopra*

The information in this section on the brain is intended to help you understand the basic functions of the brain that affect your everyday life. We will begin by reviewing the basic functions and processes of the brain as well as the role of the subconscious and unconscious. We will also dig a little deeper into the topic of consciousness, or what I call awareness. Chapter 1 will focus mostly on the malfunction of the brain: MonkeyBrain, the title of the book. Then we will look at the chemicals known as *neurotransmitters* and *hormones*. This information will help you understand the connection between the chemicals and our corresponding emotions. We will also explore the cause and the effects of *stress and fear* on our mental and physical health. Finally, we will look at techniques and exercises that enhance brain function, reduce stress, and influence emotional stability. Part I looks at some of the not so obvious things that make us sick, as well as some things that make us better.

Now let us take a brief tour of the brain and look at the basic functions and processes and how they relate to our everyday lives. The brain weighs only three pounds, yet has the capacity to hold countless memories and patterns. This extraordinary organ allows us to learn, to remember, to move, to experience the beauty of a sunset or feel emotion through the sound of music. It lets us feel the satisfaction of a great meal, the natural high from exercise, and the calm of inner peace. On the other hand, the brain can also stimulate the emotions of fear, anger, anxiety, and even insecurity. In my writing, I refer to the brain and the mind as separate. I do understand that the brain is one organ. However, I believe (as others do), that the brain does have a mind of its own. But to understand the mind, we must first understand the brain. Most neuroscientists believe that the mind is a product of the brain.[1]

---

[1]    Wang, The Neuroscience of everyday life, www.thegreatcourses.com.

We know that the mind includes awareness of self, learning, and experiences. Here we will be talking about mind and brain as it relates to awareness.

> *In order to understand mind-body medicine, we*
> *have to understand the mind; In order to understand*
> *the mind; we have to understand the brain.*
> ~ *Professor Jason M. Satterfield*

As it relates to awareness, I see the mind and brain as separate for this simple reason: the mind can be aware of what the brain is doing. It may be helpful to think of it this way: The human body is the vehicle. The brain is the engine and the mind is the driver of the vehicle. The driver controls the operations, the speed, and the direction of the vehicle and its engine. In other words, if allowed, the mind will assist and correct the brain and the physical body.

For example, let's say you're doing your weekly grocery shopping and are about to dash for the checkout, when you see a pumpkin pie. Although you are trying to lose weight and you know that you shouldn't have it, you justify it by telling yourself, "It's for my significant other." (The typical "It's for them, not for me.") But your mind knows better and reminds you that you will be tempted every time you see the pie in your refrigerator. Your mind is warning you that the temptation will probably win. You then quickly turn around and return the pie. This is the mind overriding the brain's original decision. The original decision was made by the brain based on a pattern, more than likely a conditioned pattern. In other words, you fell into a behavior that has been done many times before. The human mind gives us the opportunity to be aware and change. The brain is doing things based on chemistry, patterns, and circuits, but the mind can be the observer.

Now let's go a bit deeper. The subconscious is part of the mind and the brain. The subconscious functions within the brain and is responsible for all the involuntary automatic functions, such as breathing, perspiration, and heart and lung function. These are just some of the responsibilities of the subconscious. The subconscious is capable of fixing things that the brain is not able to do, such as physical and emotional healing. For example, if you cut yourself, the healing process is a responsibility of the subconscious. You don't have to think about the body's internal healing process. It's automatic. The entire healing process is out of our conscious control. Emotional healing is a bit different, and we will discuss this topic later. But for now, let's get back to mind versus brain. Let's go back to the reference of being cut. If you continue to have thoughts of the experience of getting cut, it is the brain reliving the memory based on a pattern. This is the MonkeyBrain reliving pain without your consent. Let's say that you are thinking about an event of the past that caused you emotional pain or stress. The thought of that event triggers the same chemicals and emotions as the original experience, such as elevating the heart rate, increasing cortisol levels, muscle tension, and perspiration. So are you choosing to relive that experience or is your brain pulling a memory file without your consent? The next time you are reliving a past experience in your head, ask yourself if you chose that memory to be recalled. Being aware of our thoughts and emotions can help us make the choice to reframe either, and can then lead us to a better emotional feeling.

Where are your thoughts most of the time? Reliving stress and fear or thinking of hope and optimism? In relation to your health, are most of your thoughts of good health or are you mostly thinking of disease and illness? Remember, your thoughts are not really happening, and you can dismiss thoughts that are not to your liking. The brain is constantly thinking. It is either reliving past experiences based on memory, solving problems, planning for the future, or even worrying about the future. Thinking is part of what the brain does. It thinks a lot! Much of this thought is of past experiences that can prevent us from forward thinking in the *now*.

As a matter of fact, an average human could have between thirty thousand to sixty thousand thoughts per day. Many of those thoughts are conscious, but how many of those thoughts are occurring unconsciously? Now, here is the dilemma: all of this thinking is not as simple as it may seem. Thoughts, emotions, and behavior are interdependent. In other words, thoughts can trigger emotions, and emotions can then influence behavior. Or emotions can trigger behavior, which in turn influences thoughts, and so on. To make matters more complicated, these three are interdependent consciously and unconsciously, resulting in unconscious thoughts, emotions, and behavior. It's no wonder we feel out of control at times. To make this easier to understand, let's look at two examples.

First we will look at a conscious positive pattern. You made a decision to make a lifestyle change to improve your health (this is the thought). Now you have a plan in your head about the positive change, which starts to make you feel better (emotion). Then you start exercising regularly and eating healthier (behavior). Here you can see how a positive thought influenced positive behavior. Now let's look at a negative unconscious pattern. You're overwhelmed with work and responsibilities, and you're feeling a bit stressed. You're worried about a work project and maybe some personal matters (thoughts). You get off work feeling too tired and unmotivated to stop at the grocery for some healthy food. Instead, you decide on a fast food drive-through (behavior). You make a reasonably healthy choice from the menu, but you also order a dessert, rewarding yourself for making it through the day (behavior). Here you can see how emotion (stress) triggered a thought process that has a negative effect on behavior and health.

These patterns should make us all question our self-awareness, especially because thoughts trigger emotions, emotions dictate our moods, and our moods influence our behavior. The good news is we can choose what we want to think about or we can allow the brain to think for itself. This leads me to the question that has boggled my mind for years. Why do we relive thoughts of pain, drama, or fear over and over? I knew that when we relive an emotionally charged thought of pain or fear, we stimulate similar if not the same chemicals as the original event. Therefore, it was obvious to me that stressful or fearful thoughts trigger the stress response, along with the corresponding stress hormones, just as in the original experience. To make matters worse, we can relive these experiences over and over in our thoughts, which, over time, disrupt the chemical balance and wreak havoc on our health as a whole.

When we allow the mind to observe our thoughts, only then can we direct the thoughts toward a better solution. We have about a ninety-second window of time to observe the thought and choose to remain in that thought and emotion or shift into another direction. Here we are talking about negative thoughts of the past or worries about the future. I am not referring to the thoughts of consciously planning your day, deciding what to wear, or solving problems. I am mostly talking about obsessively reliving stress, fear, or pain of any kind, and doubt or worry of the future. The entire thought process is driven by the communication of chemicals in the brain. They are known as *neurotransmitters.*

Understanding how the brain communicates to the body, and vice versa, can help us enhance positive experiences and reduce the negative ones.

The keys to your brain function are determined by the communication of the chemicals known as neurotransmitters and hormones. Now let's look at how this process works.

*Neurons - Synapse - Receptors - Dendrites = Communication*

## The Communication Highway of the Brain

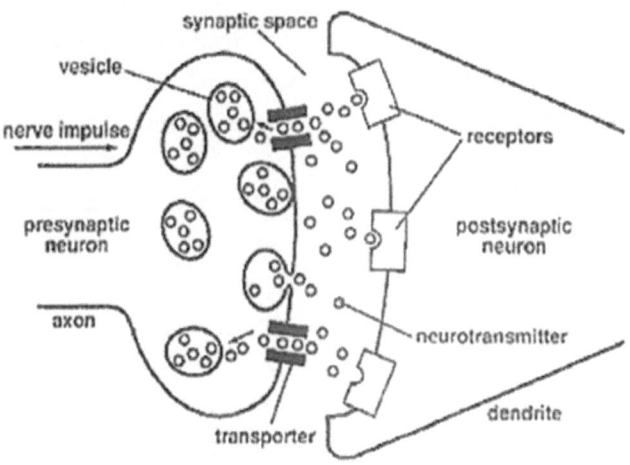

As thoughts or impulses travel from neuron to neuron in the brain, they help determine how we feel. Trillions of nerve cells, called *neurons*, are stationed throughout the body but are most highly concentrated in the brain. Neurons are connected to one another via branches called *dendrites*. These dendrites are linked together like interconnecting highways. Neurotransmitters deliver messages from one neuron to the next. The *sending* or pre-synaptic neuron produces the neurotransmitter, moving it to the *receiving* post-synaptic neuron, across a small gap called a *synapse*. Think of it as a key fitting into a lock. If it fits, the message is delivered and the *receptor* is activated. The signal then travels along the dendrites until it reaches the next synapse, where it triggers the release of more neurotransmitters. After the neurotransmitter has delivered its message, it is released from the receptor site and returns to the synapse. At this point, the neurotransmitter may be reabsorbed or just eliminated. Each neuron makes approximately one thousand synaptic connections with other neurons. There may be hundreds of trillions of synapses in the brain. These synapses are not random but form patterns that are called *circuits in the brain*. These circuits form *behavior and emotional patterns*, like tearing up over a certain song.[2] How you think and feel is affected by the activity of these circuits, which are all controlled by the intricate interaction of neurotransmitters.

Functional MRIs and PET scans now allow neuroscientists to examine brain function at many levels in real time. This has allowed for the discovery of what actions stimulate, strengthen, and regulate specific regions of the brain.

This is encouraging and important because now we can influence specific brain regions with specific actions.[3] For instance, standing on one leg, with focus and attention, balances the chemical reactions of the emotional regions of the brain known as the *hypothalamus and amygdala*. This is important because the hypothalamus and the amygdala are the brain's storage house for emotional experiences, especially painful or fearful experiences. Now let's talk about the stress response, the mechanism known as

---

2    Wang, The Neuroscience of Everyday Life, www.greatcourses.com.
3    Restak, Optimizing Brain Fitness, www.thegreatcourses.com.

the *fight-or-flight response.* These responses both trigger the release of stress hormones. Both trigger the same physiological reaction that occurs in response to a perceived harmful event or attack.

For example, if you were hiking somewhere and all of a sudden, out of the corner of your eye, you noticed a bobcat staring you down. Your fight-or-flight response would be activated. The initial reaction begins in the amygdala, which triggers a neural response in the hypothalamus. The *adrenal gland* is activated and releases a chemical known as *epinephrine,* (also known as *adrenaline*). This is followed by the release of a hormone known as *cortisol,* which increases blood pressure and blood sugar while suppressing

the immune system. This chemical reaction is what prepares us for the stress. The adrenaline provides the needed boost of energy while the additional circulation of cortisol functions to turn fatty acids into available energy. It prepares muscles throughout the body for response. Now let us go back to the story. The bobcat triggered your fight-or-flight mechanism, preparing you for the danger. You freeze at first, and hyper focus on the bobcat. You notice that it's now walking in the other direction. You then begin to feel at ease. This is partly due to the chemicals that decrease the heart rate and, consequently, the reduction in stress hormones.

This works very well for real-time danger. However, many other stressors in life can unnecessarily trigger the stress response, such as traffic, financial worries, work conditions, and even deciding what clothes to wear. And herein lies the problem. The stress response can also be activated by *merely thinking* of an event in the past that caused stress, such as a divorce, an accident, or any emotional stress or drama.

In order to understand this brain activity, we must first understand the system that controls this activity. This system is part of the central nervous system. It is known as the *autonomic nervous system*. Much of the autonomic system is out of our conscious control, such as breathing, heart rate, and digestion. The autonomic nervous system (ANS) is further divided into two systems: the *sympathetic nervous system* (SNS) raises the heart rate, and the *parasympathetic nervous system* (PNS) lowers the heart rate.[4] To make this easier to understand, the systems will be defined this way: *warming* for the SNS system that raises the heart rate, and *cooling* for the PNS system that lowers the heart rate. We will get deeper into this system later, but for now, let's look at how memory works and the connection between memory, emotions, and behavior.

First, let's look at what is known as *emotional memory*. Although the science of how and where the brain decides to store most memory is unknown, we do know some things for sure. The latest neuroscience has shown that we do store experiences of fear or pain in the emotional regions of the brain for the long term. This is also called *emotional memory*. *Long-term memory* is stored for many years and, in most cases, a lifetime. A very sad example of long-term negative emotional memory would be the memory of the death of a family member or good friend. Another example would be a very traumatic event, such as an automobile accident, a divorce, or a soldier's combat experience. Those memories can last for life. They are also the memories that tend to pop up in our thoughts at the will of the brain (in the unconscious) or MonkeyBrain.

Some of these unconscious negative emotional memories (out of our conscious control or not purposefully remembered) are automatic, such as when the brain memorizes how to ride a

---

[4]    Wang, The Neuroscience of Everyday Life, www.thegreatcourses.com.

bicycle; you don't have to think about it. This memory is also known as *implicit memory*. When we experience a very emotional event, the brain records not only the details of the experience, (where, when, what happened, who was there, etc.), but also the emotions that we experienced at the time of the event. The entire memory of an emotional event (a car accident, a death, a combat situation, a wedding, etc.) is remembered by two systems in the brain and stored in two separate areas of the brain. The brain has specific areas in which information is stored or that operate specific areas of the body.

For example, the left side of the brain contains language capability, while the right side holds pictures as well as the ability to view objects in space. Memory for faces is located in the right side of the brain, while the name of the individual is located in the left side of the brain. This is why we can recognize an old friend almost immediately, but the brain may require several seconds to recall their name.

The old saying that we only use 10 percent of our brain is just a myth. We use the entire brain at all times, and the left and right are always communicating and conveying information and signals back and forth. Studies tell us that we can have two types of memory for the same situation, especially if the experience is associated with strong emotions.[5] A single experience of a traumatic event or a very happy event with strong emotions can leave a detailed memory of the experience and a memory of the emotions connected to the experience. This emotional memory contains the memory of the physiological response at the time of the experience. This physiological response (fight-or-flight or stress response) can include muscle tension, increased heart rate, rapid

---

[5]    Satterfield, Mind-Body Medicine, www.thegreatcourses.com.

breathing, anxiety, and other reactions associated with fear, terror, fright, or joy. When we remember traumatic or horrible events, the brain often recalls both the details and the emotional memory at the same time. This means that when we are thinking of a traumatic event from the past, we will also experience the feelings we had at that time, such as increased heart rate, desperation, and panic. The brain has the ability to recall the details and the emotions of an experience on purpose or by accident. This means that we do not have to consciously think of the experience. This memory can also be recalled by the brain at any time.

The brain also has the ability to recall one part of the memory without the other. We can also have an experience that prompts an emotional memory but does not bring up the details of that memory. For instance, you may be driving to work, minding your own business, and all of a sudden, you feel your mood change. Your mood becomes gloomy for no apparent reason. What may have happened is this: your brain noticed a car, a location, or a song on the radio that may have triggered a memory file that had a negative emotion attached to it. The emotion of the old memory file was triggered without the details. Now you are experiencing the emotion but don't really know why. How many times have you heard someone say, "I woke up on the wrong side of the bed today"? Could it be because that person had dreams the night before that triggered chemicals and negative emotions? Since emotions, thoughts, and behavior are interdependent, it is possible. We will look at this connection later on, but let us continue on with how memory works. For now, we know that negative or positive emotional memory can be automatic and long-term.

On the other hand, basic information and knowledge is stored as *short-term memory* and is known as *explicit memory*. Short-term memory can be stored for seconds to years and is processed through the *hippocampus*. It is usually information without emotional attachment, such as trivial facts, telephone numbers, and most general information. For example, remembering facts such as the year Abraham Lincoln served as president or remembering a telephone number. As it relates to short-term memory, repetition or the value that we place on the information and/or an experience determines if it is stored for just a few seconds, days, or even years. For instance, if you were introduced to a group of people by name and you had to recall the names a few hours later, you may only remember a few of the names easily. If you were asked to recall the names after a week, you may not remember any of the names. This is partly because the brain has to sift through information, lots of it, and similar to a computer, it has to store some things in what I call junk files. These memories can be very difficult to retrieve.[6]

But we will usually remember the experiences that we value, such as the names of people who impressed us or maybe attracted us in some way. The impression or the attraction created the value that encouraged the brain to store it in a way that allows it to be recalled easily. In addition, association can be used to increase the chances of retrieval. For example, if you want to remember someone's name, associate it with an object, another person, or an event with emotional attachment. This will provide two references for that memory file, which allows the memory to be retrieved much easier.

How many books have you read but of which you don't remember many of the details? We can read an entire book and yet are unable to retrieve certain character names or the totality of the

---

[6]     Restak, Optimizing Brain Fitness, www.thegreatcourses.com

story. We do remember that we enjoyed it or didn't like it. We know that it all goes in, but we just can't retrieve all of it.

Unfortunately, emotional memory that has pain and fear attached to it is stored in the long-term regions: the amygdala and hypothalamus. Many things, such as a scent, a song, a location, or even a meal, could trigger a memory that can pop up at any time, for many years. Reliving this emotional pain and fear is MonkeyBrain. The brain dictates our daily experiences at every level, from breathing and sleeping, to learning, making decisions, and even loving or hating.

Neuroscience is starting to provide explanations for every aspect of behavior.[7] As a result, we can now see the connection between thoughts, emotions, and behavior.[8] We are also understanding how negative emotional memory (negative thoughts of the past or fear of the future) contributes to more negative emotions and to more negative behavior. Understanding how memory works can help us improve positive experiences and reduce the negative ones. In order to improve emotions and behavior, we must first improve the thoughts. In other words, if we are reliving a memory that was fearful, painful, or stressful, we will also trigger the release of the stress hormones that can and will make us sick. Patrolling our thoughts and reframing negative thoughts into positive ones are sure ways to improve our emotions, and, more important, our overall health. Just keep this triangle in mind. Thoughts trigger emotions and emotions influence behavior. Emotions trigger behavior that influences thoughts, and behavior can trigger thoughts that influence emotions. These three are interdependent and always influence each other.

---

[7]    Wang, The Neuroscience of Everyday Life, www.thegreatcourses.com.

[8]    Satterfield, Mind-Body Medicine, www.thegreatcourses.com.

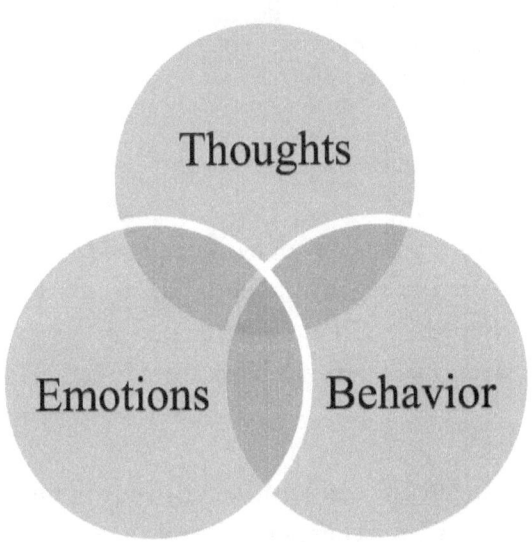

The brain is forever changing, and when we discover the evolution of those changes, we can and should adapt and influence the health of our brains. We know that exercising the brain (brain training) improves memory and many other functions of the brain. We also know that exercising the physical body (physical fitness) improves the health and function of the body. Now we also know that certain activities and exercising the physical body with specific movement helps regulate the balance of brain chemistry while strengthening the systems within the brain. Therefore, a healthier body equals a healthier brain, and vice versa. The brain and the body are interconnected, and as we integrate the conditioning programs together, we enhance the functions of the brain as well as the health and functions of the body.

Now let's get a better understanding of the subconscious and the unconscious. Here, we will look at the roles and the responsibilities of each. The brain operates consciously, unconsciously, and subconsciously, independently and simultaneously. I know this sounds complicated, but the following explanation will help you better understand their functions within the brain.

## Subconscious

Although at this point we aren't sure if the subconscious is located in a specific region of the brain, we do know that it functions within the brain and throughout the entire body. The subconscious has many responsibilities and functions within the brain.

From the moment you are born, it runs your brain and bodily functions without your conscious control. It regulates all of the intricate processes of digestion and elimination, as in bowel movements and urination. When not opposed, it has absolute control of the silent involuntary functions, such as the actions of the heart, the circulation of blood, the functions of the lungs, and other internal organs. Also the subconscious regulates the intricate functions of all human cells.

Basically, the subconscious controls all of the automatic functions, (out of our conscious control) of our brain and body. This includes spontaneous emotional reactions, such as crying, laughing, loving, or hating, regardless of whether they are logical or illogical. But despite its lack of logic and reasoning, the subconscious is the most powerful driving force in our actions.

These actions and reactions are the result of programming by our parents, teachers, religion, politics, and society. This programming becomes emotionally powerful memories and creates the blueprints that become the basis for unconscious behavior, such as, low self-esteem, anxiety, or a positive outlook on life. This behavior is conditioned and becomes part of our personalities. Subconscious programming is not right or wrong; it is just the content that you have been programmed with, and with work or with conscious effort, it can be changed. The subconscious does not operate in the context of time and does not recognize past or future.

The subconscious just is. It perceives by intuition. And when encouraged (exercise, balanced nutrition, and sleep), it heals the body and keeps it balanced. We must condition the subconscious just like we train the brain or work the body. However, the conditioning of the subconscious is very specific, and those specific exercises will be provided in Part III. But for now, let us continue our tour of the brain. Let's move on to the unconscious.

## Unconscious

The unconscious can be a bit misleading because we can be knocked out unconscious with no awareness, or we can be unconscious and awake. In other words, we can be on autopilot. Here, we will be talking about what is known as the cognitive unconscious. It is also known as the autopilot. It is when you are driving your car while listening to the radio and maybe talking with a fellow passenger. Your brain is basically unconscious during this time and returns to full awareness only when you sense danger or see a red light. This is why we can drive for miles, arrive at our destination, and yet barely remember details of the drive. The main part of our mental processing takes place in the unconscious. The brain shifts from conscious to unconscious many times throughout our day. This is when the brain rebuilds, repairs, and consolidates memory. The brain is still thinking and running your body in the unconscious, but the thinking is being done by the brain and not you.

For instance, if you are doing a routine task and you are thinking about the task at hand, that is you doing the thinking. If you are doing the task but thinking about what happened yesterday or worrying about tomorrow, that is your brain doing the thinking. The brain is basically pulling memory files without your consent. The brain is constantly pulling memories for reference to make sense of the stimuli that comes in by way of our senses. Remember, pain and fear patterns have emotional attachment and therefore deeper connections. These deep connections and circuits tend to be recalled in the cognitive unconscious very easily. This is why we tend to relive emotional pain and fear over and over, consciously and unconsciously. Now let us move on to Chapter 1, MonkeyBrain. Here we will explore the meaning behind the title and why I consider it a malfunction of the brain.

# Chapter 1

# The MonkeyBrain

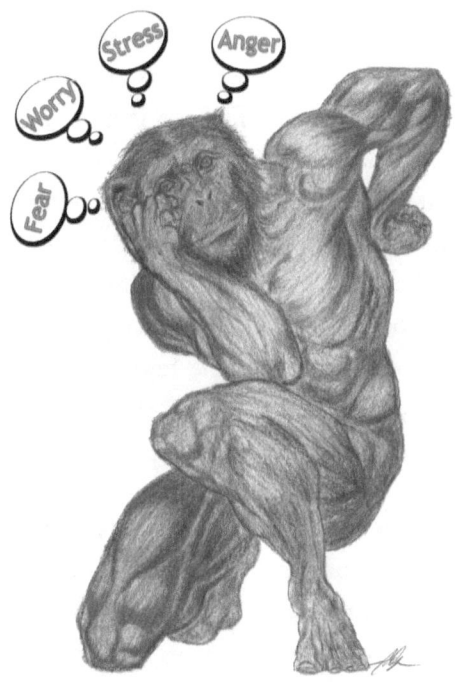

*If we don't consciously select where we want to go, we go where
the unconscious wants us to go. Until we make the unconscious,
conscious, it will select our lives and we will just call it fate.
So in that regard, most of us are on automatic pilot.*
*~ Carl Jung*

You have heard me mention MonkeyBrain earlier, including the
title; and now we will explore the meaning. The MonkeyBrain is
a state of mind. It is when the brain is compulsively thinking of
a past event that caused emotional pain, such as grief, jealousy,

resentment, or pain of any kind. This includes worry, doubt, or fear of the future. The MonkeyBrain shows itself in many ways. This includes our daily interactions with others and ourselves. I will define the MonkeyBrain as *me* or *I*, or *my story*. It's the voice in our head that says: That is mine, I am stronger, I am better, I am smarter, I'm not good enough, or you betrayed *me*, you did *me* wrong, you hurt *my* feelings and on and on. The *me* or *I* is also known as the ego. The ego is that voice in our head, and that voice is the MonkeyBrain. Oh, that voice! At times, the voices are very loud and arrogant, and other times soft but painful. It is the internal brain chatter that is always creating an inner dialogue of chaos. This voice is the incessant stream of brain chatter, the memories that the brain recalls in the unconscious. Most neuroscientists agree that the brain is in the unconscious up to 80 percent of the time for most of us. This means that we can be unconscious, operating on autopilot, for most of our day.[9]

As was mentioned in Part I, the main part of our mental processing takes place in the unconscious. The brain shifts from conscious to unconscious any time it can. It is the only way for the brain to catch up on all the work that needs to be done. The brain needs plenty of time to consolidate all of the input, and does its work in the unconscious. It is also when the brain chatter, or what I call the MonkeyBrain, comes out full force. The brain loves to shift into the unconscious while we are doing our routine tasks, like brushing our teeth or driving to work. How many times have you pulled into your work parking lot and barely remember the drive. This is partly because your brain was on autopilot or unconscious for part of the drive. You were only forced into full consciousness when your eyes saw a red light, heard a horn, or sensed danger. During this time, when we are

---

9    Wang, The Neuroscience of Everyday Life, www.thegreatcourses.com

operating on autopilot, the MonkeyBrain loves to come out and play. Remember, the MonkeyBrain recalls everything that we experience that is of pain. It includes legitimate and psychological pain and fear (emotional memory). Let me remind you that most stressful thoughts are attached to pain and fear in some way. Emotional memory resides in our thoughts. These thoughts are not really happening, but thinking so can make it feel that way.

You may be asking now, "Is It possible to get rid of this inner voice?" The answer is no. However, we can reduce the brain chatter and change the content. It is also why this voice has been called the pain ego. I first learned of this from the book *A New Earth*, written by *Eckart Tolle*. Tolle identifies this voice as the pain ego since it is the inner dialog that loves to relive pain, drama, or trauma of any kind.[10] Tolle's book changed my way of thinking so much. I recommend that you read it. I was unaware that I could choose to change the content of my brain's chatter. After learning this, I was then able to allow the voice to be heard and could make a conscious choice to bring myself back to the moment by shifting to another thought or mood that I wanted to have. This shifting is also known as reframing or reappraisal.

For example, one day, I was reliving an emotional experience in my head that was causing me to feel bad. I call this story *MonkeyBrain in the Rain*. My brain was reliving an emotional experience that caused me heartache. I felt wronged, and I just wanted to tell the person what I was feeling. In this case, there was no communication and therefore no closure. My thoughts were completely ego driven, and I just wanted the other person to feel the same pain that I was experiencing. Once I became aware that my brain was obsessing, I literally told myself to stop it, to

---

[10]   Tolle, A New Earth, 129.

shut up. This glimpse of awareness allowed me to just be in the moment, the present, outside of my thoughts. On this particular day, it was raining very hard, and I put all of my attention on the rain and the sound. For a few minutes, I just listened to the sound and watched the drops fall. I was outside my MonkeyBrain the entire time—no thoughts of the emotional memory. As a matter of fact, I had no thoughts at all, just the sound of the rain. It was just peaceful being in that moment. Unfortunately, as soon as I took my attention away from the rain just for a split second, my MonkeyBrain pulled me back into the drama, and once again, I was reliving that painful experience. It was like a wild monkey swinging from limb to limb, pulling another painful emotion with each swing. But I pulled myself back to the moment again, focused on the rain, and again, I was out of my thinking brain and the emotional pain. Thinking and talking about our problems is our greatest addiction, and that addiction can be just as harmful to our health as any other,

This experience proved to me that we can choose to get out of our emotional pain by being in the present, and that alone stops the brain from thinking about the painful or stressful situation. I learned that I had the control to patrol the inner dialogue in my head, and I slowly began to change the chatter's content. We must first become aware of the thoughts in our head, because then we can patrol what the brain is thinking about. This simple awareness that the brain's chatter was just that, brain chatter based on memory, allowed me to hear the chatter for what it was and to make a conscious choice to change the content. If I were having a thought of something that I didn't want, such as, stress, resentment, or failure, I just began to think of what I did want. For example, if a thought arises of a past event that caused stress, we can choose to direct the next thought to the solution of that stressful event.

Although we cannot change the past event, we can now change the way we think and feel about it. This inner dialogue is much different than being in a situation where the chaos is being caused by another person or an outside source, such as an angry spouse or child or annoying co-worker. This is just letting someone or something suck you into their pain and drama, and it happens all of the time. There are some people who are stuck in their MonkeyBrain, always thinking and sharing negative information or creating and causing more stress for themselves. Some people will try to pull you into their pain, drama, and stress. You can avoid this by just being non-reactive. So long as you do not identify with their pain or engage in the conversation, you can avoid being sucked in. We can be empathetic without identifying with their emotions. You can just listen and not react, and this alone will shrink their MonkeyBrain and yours as well. In some cases, non-reaction to the other could inflame the situation. This is usually due to the other's needs to fuel their addiction to stress. Chapter 4 will provide you with more specifics on stress addiction.

I devoted an entire chapter to stress because I believe that fear and stress create serious chemical imbalances, causing health issues and emotional instability. If the other person is stressed more often than not, their brain is likely to be addicted to the chemicals driven by the stress response, such as adrenaline. Their brain's addiction to stress will look for anything that stimulates adrenalin.

Arguing or disagreements are a sure way to stimulate stress hormones (adrenalin, and cortisol) while depleting the rewarding chemicals that affect our mood and motivation (serotonin and dopamine). In these cases, it's probably best to remove yourself from the situation as soon as possible.

If you pay attention to the way that you feel the next time you have an argument or disagreement, you will feel the adrenalin. The adrenalin is just part of the body's stress response, and it is our warning to back off. The brain actually becomes very addicted to adrenalin. This is precisely why we can fall into patterns of arguments with others that really have nothing to do with the real problem. We are affected by other people's energy and their pain and drama. If we are not totally conscious and aware, we can easily be sucked right into their world.

We all have it, this mind chatter, and we cannot get rid of it; we can only shrink it by being in the present. We cannot be in the MonkeyBrain and the present at the same time. It is not possible. When we are in the now, the present, we are not thinking; we are observing. This includes the negative self-talk in your head. Ignore it; don't give it any fuel and it will slowly but surely shrink. Any time the MonkeyBrain arises, be aware and bring yourself back to the moment. Reframe your next thought and begin to think thoughts of what you do want. That simple awareness will pull you away from the negative thought, and you will avoid the emotion that would have followed. This includes repeat situations that relationships tend to fall into.

For example, your child or significant other constantly leaves their clothes or shoes in the middle of the floor. Your aggravation triggers the angry stress response, which will eventually be the way that you react to that situation every time. Practice non-reaction, and even those repeat situations are changed. It is really just behavior and emotional patterns that are conditioned over time.

Brain patterns are basically brain habits. Stress patterns can also become habits. This includes traffic, disagreements, or worrying.

All of these examples stimulate the release of dopamine, adrenalin, and cortisol. If you don't allow yourself to complete the fight-or-flight cycle, you will remain in stress mode.[11] More details will follow in Chapter 4 on the different stages of stress and how it affects our health.

The practice of non-reaction and remaining in the present can become an addiction as well. The brain will become addicted to the positive rewarding chemicals and hormones that are triggered by peace and calm. And there you have it: a positive addiction is formed.

But the most important thing to remember is that the MonkeyBrain only lives through negativity and problems. It is fueled by reliving painful, fearful, or traumatic experiences with others or in one's head. If you pay close attention to your conversations with others, you will notice the MonkeyBrain in yourself or in the other person. Remember, the MonkeyBrain loves negative content. This includes complaining, blaming, and judging. Most conversations tend to have some negative content. We love to share our bad day, our terrible story, and our physical pain. It is just because most of us are conditioned from a young age to share our day, especially the bad parts of the day, or what we perceive to be bad.

First, most of us are conditioned wrong to begin with, and then we develop a stress response that forms a pattern and a connection. The brain now slowly becomes addicted to the chemicals driven by the stress response, and the brain seeks that connection again. Once you have relived a stressful or fearful experience in your head just a few times, a behavioral circuit in the brain is formed, and a bad habit of *stinking thinking* has made its connection. Now the

---

[11]    Wang, The Neuroscience of Everyday Life, Lecture 15.

brain begins to crave the chemical and begins to seek out stinking thinking for relief. It is a common problem in today's society. The brain's patterns are very strong, and without mindful, conscious effort, and sometimes even actions, the brain's faulty pattern will win. In other words, the brain is just a machine following instructions that have been conditioned over time and which the mind can override. Remember the analogy: the automobile is the body, the engine is the brain, and the driver of the automobile is the mind. The mind can steer the brain in the right direction.

For example, a habit of negative thinking is a conditioned pattern of the brain. When you are aware of the negative thought and redirect the thought to a positive thought, this is a mindful, conscious effort that replaces the negative pathway into a positive one. Let's say you were dealing with a stressful situation that is out of your control. You dealt with the problem as best you could but you were still feeling a bit stressed. You decide to take a walk or run, or you hit the gym for a workout. This is a mindful, conscious action. The chemicals triggered by this action help reduce the stress hormones, and that will help you think less of the stressful situation. This is precisely why I use physical fitness to shrink the MonkeyBrain. Remember, the MonkeyBrain is stress, fear, pain, and drama. We already know that physical exercise has been proven to reduce stress and anxiety, so why not use it.

Legitimate stress and psychological stress (emotional memories) are both reduced by the chemicals that are stimulated by physical exercise. Active living is no longer a luxury; it is a necessity for emotional survival. In other words, movement of the body triggers the release of neurotransmitters and hormones that help reduce stress hormones, increase chemicals that improve one's mood, and help to regulate the balance. Once you have developed a positive habit of exercise for some time, the brain will slowly but surely get addicted to the rewarding chemicals that are stimulated. Here is how I look at it: we all have some habits that are considered to be bad, and we have habits that are considered to be good. Take a look at how you feel in the good and bad situations. Consider losing some of the bad habits and replacing them with good habits. The best way to trump a bad habit is to override it with three good habits.

All of the things that we do become habits, and eventually the brain will store a pattern and connection for that habit. The same applies to exercise. It stimulates a number of rewarding and feel-good chemicals, and the brain will look for that connection as well. And there you have it: a positive addiction to exercise is formed. The goal is to create as many positive and constructive habits as possible. All habits do count, even the small habits, such as making your bed, thinking optimistically, being compassionate, and drinking water.

Then there are the habits that I consider to be the most important, such as awareness of our ego, the habit of being grateful, the habit of non-judgment, the habit of loving, and the habit of accepting the things that we can't change. We can choose to be addicted to the MonkeyBrain (fear, stress, doubt, anger, resentment, jealousy, impatience, and intolerance), or we can choose to be addicted to being good to ourselves, kind and helpful to others, compassionate, and confident. Use as many positive habits as it takes to shrink the MonkeyBrain. And remember, the fastest way to cage the monkey is to be in the present. It is our choice. Focus your thoughts at the level of the solution instead of thinking at the level of the problem. Think of what you *do want* instead of what you *do not want*.

We cannot change the past; we can only change our attitudes, and that will change the future. I'm going to share with you my own personal MonkeyBrain story and how I reframed the thoughts that eventually reduced the stress and fear, and ultimately changed the outcome completely. This is just one example. However, this experience enabled me to utilize a stress reduction technique that I have used with clients in the past. I call this technique *intentional shifting,* and the process usually begins with some physical movements, such as walking. This time, however, I couldn't use physical activity to make the immediate shift in chemistry; I could only mentally shift my way out of the stress. This story is so profound that if I hadn't written it down, I wouldn't even believe it. But I did, and here it is.

The name of this story is "MonkeyBrain in the Airplane." It is a great example of being aware of stress and making a choice to change the emotion regarding the stressful situation. Those of us who are religiously inclined would just consider this prayer: To ask, believe, and receive. Now here is how the story goes.

The Joyefit Team and I organize and facilitate wellness and adventure retreats in Costa Rica. The retreat includes accommodations and a private chef that prepares a special menu designed for body improvement. Much time was spent beforehand coordinating the menu with the chef. Everything was approved and accepted by him two days prior to my arrival to Costa Rica.

While waiting at the airport terminal for my flight to board, I received a message from the chef. It said: "I have a family emergency and will not be able to cook for your group. I'm sorry." All of my alarms went off. What was I going to do? How was I going to find another chef in a foreign country in such little time? My MonkeyBrain went ballistic, and as usual, made me start thinking of the worst possible scenario. My palms began to sweat, my heart rate increased, I was in full-blown fight-or-flight with nowhere to run and no one to fight.

Thankfully, the passengers were called for boarding and my brain had to shift focus and pay attention to boarding the flight. The MonkeyBrain was put on hold while I boarded the plane, found my assigned seat, and strapped myself in for takeoff. Remember, the MonkeyBrain is always put on hold when you focus on the moment. Within seconds of fastening my seatbelt, my MonkeyBrain took over my thoughts again, full force, reminding me I had twelve guests that would have to be fed for seven days, and I had no chef!

I was so stressed and worried that I was literally shaking. I knew I had to shift my emotions because the feeling that I was having was not good for me or the situation.

I decided to use the intentional shifting technique. This technique is designed to slowly change your emotions about a stressful situation. In neuroscience, it is called *reappraisal.* The process is very simple; all that you need is a pen and paper and your imagination. Here is the actual copy of the process.

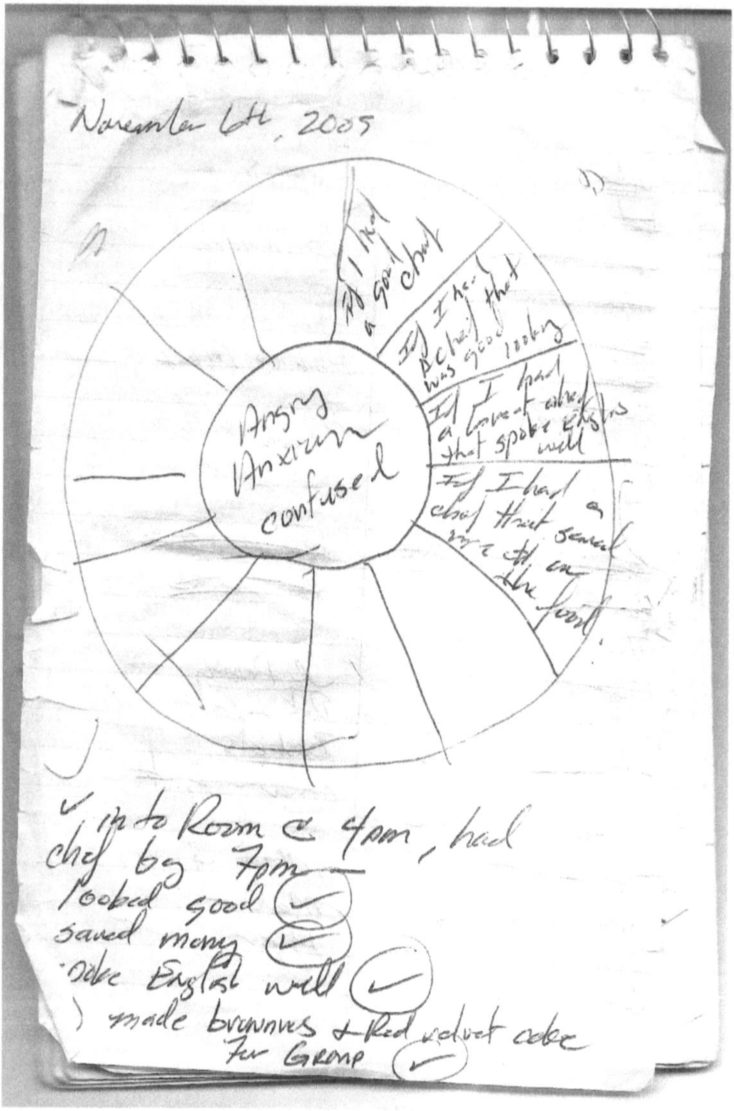

November 6th, 2005

Angry
Anxious
confused

If I had a good chef

If I had A chef that was good looking

If I had a cove of cake that spoke English well

If I had a chef that served more ... on the front.

✓ up to Room @ 4pm, had
chef by 7pm —
looked good ✓
saved money ✓
spoke English well ✓
) made brownies + Red velvet cake
for Group ✓

You start by drawing a circle about the size of a silver dollar in the center of the page. Inside the circle, you write how you are feeling about the situation. In my case, I was feeling angry, anxious, and confused.

Now that you are clear about your feelings, you draw a large circle around the small circle, similar to a donut.

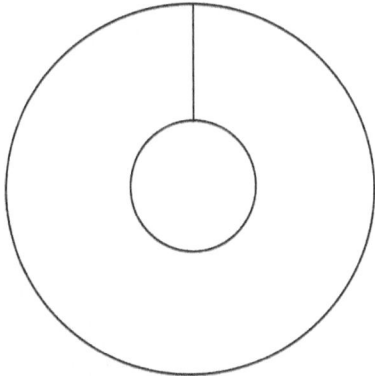

In the outer circle, you draw straight lines toward the outside of the circle to make at least six separate areas. This will leave you

with separate areas in the outer circle to write. Here is where you have to use your imagination. Since you cannot change the circumstance, the goal is to feel better about the situation.

Now you begin the writing process of what would make you feel a little better about the situation.

Now in my case, the first feel-better statement was "I would feel better if I had a chef." That didn't make me feel any better. So I continued to write more statements that would make me feel better. My next feel-better statements were "If I had a chef that was good-looking" and "If I had a chef that spoke English well," both of which made me feel a little better. At this point, my stress level had started to go down and I did feel better, so I wrote one more feel-good statement: "If I had a chef that saved me money on the food." Now that statement really made feel good!

After writing and imagining all of my statements, I did feel better about the situation and actually fell asleep for most of the flight. The plane landed in Costa Rica, and I continued on in a vehicle for the four-hour ride to the resort location, with not one thought or worry about the chef situation during the drive.

I reached my destination at 4 p.m. and began to check into my hotel for the night. The group of twelve was to arrive at noon the following day, and I had just a few hours to secure a chef. Apparently, my brain believed my feel-better statements and did not remind me of the chef situation until now. As the front desk attendant was handing me the room key, another hotel employee greeted me by name. I didn't really remember him until he introduced himself and reminded me of the white-water rafting tour that he had helped me organize.

His name was Paco. We spoke for a few minutes about some new tours that he could help me with, and I began to think of the chef situation. At this point, I had nothing to lose, so I asked him if he could find a chef for me. He smiled and replied, "Of course I can help you. My family owns a restaurant, and I am a chef. The name of the restaurant is Munchados (which means Munchies in English)." After telling him I was interested, Paco said, "Go ahead and check into your room and relax. I will come up to your room when I get off at 7 p.m. to discuss the details of my service." He arrived promptly at 7 p.m., we discussed my needs, and went over the menu. He gave me the cost, which was $400 less than the other chef! Paco presented himself very well and had a good command of the English language.

Now take a brief look at my original intentional shifting page, at my feel-better statements. Paco exceeded all my wishes, including a gorgeous assistant who happened to be his wife. So to recap the MonkeyBrain fix: I arrived at 4 p.m. and secured a good-looking chef who spoke English well and saved me money, all by 7 p.m.! It was the first time that I had used this technique on myself, and I could not believe what had happened. Paco and his wife served us amazing food, with great communication and style. In addition, they allowed the guests to help and learn how to prepare some of the meals. To this day, I still use Paco and his wife because of their excellent service.

I received what I intended, plus more! It made me realize, without a doubt, the power of intentions and forcing the brain to think about the solution instead of being stuck in the problem. Or was there more to it (answered prayer or both)? Just remember, being mindful of the solution to whatever the problem is, and adding some conscious action of shifting, you can fake your way out of a negative emotion. Always think of what you *do want* instead of what you *do not want.* You will be amazed to see how your life will change when you learn to redirect mismanaged imagination. Negative thinking (MonkeyBrain) is a habit that can be broken. Try to recognize and catch the first thought that started the negative compulsive thinking. If possible, take a walk or take ten deep breaths to clear your head. Accept it for what it is: just thought. Redirect the next few thoughts to anything positive, and then begin to think of the solution to the problem that started the negative stream of thoughts. Write down as many solutions to the problem that would make you feel better, and don't stop writing until you do feel better about the situation. If the thought pops up again, keep redirecting toward the solution and press on with your day. Be present in all of your activities, and stay out of your head. Consciously direct your thoughts to what you are doing at each moment.

> *"Yesterday is history, tomorrow is a mystery, today is the present, and that is why it is called a gift."*
> *~ Unknown*

Now before we move on to Chapter 2, let us review Chapter 1. The MonkeyBrain rules when the brain is obsessively thinking about a past event that caused fear, drama, trauma, or stress. The MonkeyBrain also loves to worry, doubt, and stress about the future. And don't forget the thoughts and feelings of failure, inferiority, and low self-esteem, or superiority, judgment, and anger. All are alibis for the MonkeyBrain. The MonkeyBrain always thinks of the worst-case scenario. Techniques and/or exercises to tame the MonkeyBrain will be provided in chapters to come. Sometimes we need an arsenal to cage the monkey. Use as many coping techniques as needed.

Now we can move forward to chapter 2: specifics on brain chemistry and how it relates to our everyday lives.

CHAPTER 2

# Brain Chemistry

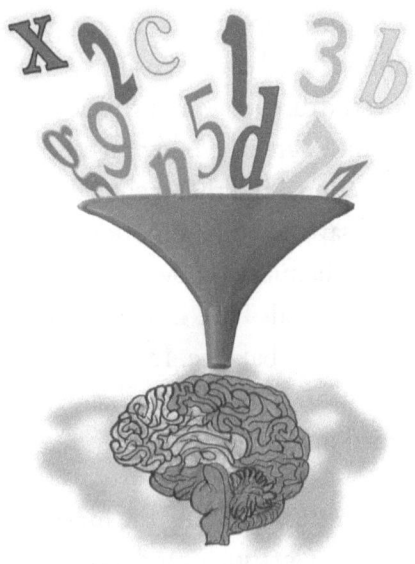

*The brain's chemistry determines how we*
*feel, how we speak, and how we act.*

As I was doing the research for this book, I discovered much
more than I had anticipated. I expected to find the obvious: that
exercise and proper nutrition have positive and regulating effects
on brain chemistry. To my surprise, I learned that everything that
we do has some effect on the balance of our brain chemistry. And I
mean everything. Brain chemistry determines the communication
between the brain and the body, and vice versa. These chemicals
are known as neurotransmitters and hormones.[12]

---

[12]    Wang, The Neuroscience of Everyday Life, www.thegreatcourses.com

Communication is a two-way street; information comes in via sensory input (hearing, seeing, touching, tasting, and smelling). The brain reacts to the body's sensory inputs by sending commands back into the body that connect, improve, protect, or react in some way, resulting in an effort to balance the whole. This is also true of sheer thought in the brain, such as anger, grief, joy, and hope. Sheer thought can be based on real or imaginary thinking. The brain doesn't know the difference and will act accordingly until it is analyzed by the mind and the body together. All of our senses trigger chemical reactions, and that includes emotionally charged thoughts. Yes, I did say thoughts. Emotionally charged thoughts also stimulate these chemicals known as neurotransmitters and hormones. These chemicals have important responsibilities and help maintain brain/body balance. In some cases, however, over- or underproduction of any one of these chemicals can cause health issues and emotional instability.

The stress hormone *cortisol* is among the most important because of its critical functions. Cortisol is produced by the adrenal cortex in response to stress and also when we have low blood sugar. The primary function of cortisol is to increase blood sugar to normal healthy levels, as it aids in fat, protein, and carbohydrate metabolism. However, overproduction of cortisol due to overeating sugars and starches or stress can disrupt the balance, causing blood sugar imbalance and circulatory issues. And if that isn't bad enough, overproduction of cortisol causes additional storage of *body fat* (adipose tissue) in the belly region. *Stress gets us high and it makes us fat!* To make matters worse, high levels can suppress the immune system and decrease bone formation as well. In today's society, we are bombarded with stressors, such as traffic, work, and financial issues, from which we cannot escape. We remain stuck in the fight-or-flight. We then remain in a heightened stress mode, causing a prolonged release of *epinephrine* a.k.a. *adrenalin*, and *cortisol* while increasing the heart rate.

On the other hand, we also have stress-reducing neurotransmitters, such as acetylcholine, *serotonin, GABA*, and *oxytocin,* as well as *vasopressin* in men. These neurotransmitters are recuperative. They slow down the heart rate and affect our moods. Of all of the chemicals that help lower the heart rate, oxytocin and vasopressin are especially important for shutting down the stress hormones that raise the heart rate. Until not so long ago, oxytocin was known for its role in sexual reproduction, in particular during and after childbirth, maternal bonding, and breast feeding. However, recent research has shown a number of other activities that stimulate the release of this stress-reducing hormone. Oxytocin functions as a neurotransmitter and a hormone, which gives this chemical additional influence on reducing and even inhibiting the release of stress hormones. Now that we know what activities stimulate oxytocin, we can use them as additional tools to reduce stress and tension in ways that were not known in the past. The scientific research indicates promising data that demonstrates the powerful positive effect that oxytocin has on the central nervous system. We will look at specific activities and behavior that activate the release of this chemical later, but for now, let's move on.

All of these chemicals and hormones determine how we feel, whether it is input from our sensory system (real-time events) or just thoughts. In other words, good experiences and good thoughts can stimulate rewarding, positive chemicals and reduce the stress hormones, allowing us to feel good. On the other hand, stressful, fearful, or painful events or thoughts stimulate stress hormones and reduce or deplete the feel-good chemicals that will make us feel bad. If you pay close attention the next time that you are thinking about a positive or negative past experience, you may notice the chemical shift. How did you feel during and after the thought? If the thought made you feel bad, now is the time to shift to another thought until the feeling changes.

Now let's look at some of the things that we do and how they influence our chemical balance and our emotions. For instance, listening to soothing music or watching a beautiful sunset can stimulate chemicals known as *dopamine* and *serotonin*, which allows us to feel calm, relaxed, and a bit in awe. This is because dopamine is the main reward or pleasure chemical and it gives us a little boost of energy, while serotonin brings it back down to allow us to feel calm and relaxed. Dopamine is the main driver for increasing the heart rate, and is also responsible for the affective component of memory, which makes you believe that the event is worthwhile enough to reserve a sufficient amount of space in the brain where memories are stored. Just think about your most vivid memories, such as 9/11. You probably remember where you were, what time it was, who you were with, as well as the emotions of the experience. The shock of this event triggered the stress response and the release of dopamine, which created the value for the brain to store the memory of that event.

*Acetylcholine,* on the other hand, is the main driver for decreasing the heart rate. For example, if we witness an accident, the brain instantly releases a bit of dopamine, adrenaline, and cortisol, preparing the body to deal with whatever stress comes our way. The release of dopamine and adrenaline gives us a boost of energy and makes us very alert. This is because dopamine is also the primary fight-or-flight neurotransmitter. Adrenaline drives us away from the danger as cortisol prepares the body for the stress by releasing more sugar into the bloodstream. Once we get away from the accident, the brain releases a bit of acetylcholine, serotonin, and *GABA,* which lowers the heart rate and reduces the stress hormones. This is an example of a complete stress response cycle. However, if you continued to think about the accident, the chemicals that bring the heart rate down would not be activated, leaving you stressed out!

Every experience we have stimulates a chemical reaction in the brain that determines the way we feel. These chemicals perceive everything that we are and everything that we know while instantly conveying information from the brain throughout the rest of the body. For example, exercise stimulates dopamine as the reward, noradrenaline for motivation, and a bit of serotonin to enhance our mood. This communication of chemicals happens to us hundreds of thousands of times a day. Every breath we take, every thought we have, everything that we eat or drink, every conversation we have, and even reading these words stimulates the release of certain chemicals. We react to everything that comes into our bodies by way of our sensory system, our senses.

We also have senses that are inner processes of the brain, such as intuition, inspiration, and premonition. This is also known as the *sixth sense*, and is the internal sense that is not stimulated from the outside but is our inner guidance sense. Call it what you may: a gut feeling, a vibe, intuition, premonition, or even inspiration. This sense triggers a chemical reaction as well. When we are aware, we feel it. To feel without the use of the physical senses is remarkable, and this needs more study. I believe the evidence is overwhelming and deserves more attention.

Thanks to the brain's remarkable ability to instantly adapt to our ever-changing environment, such as weather, the energy of other people, a traffic accident, or our environment, we make tiny corrections to our chemistry by way of *intuitive reactions.* Otherwise we wouldn't make it through a day alive. In most cases, the brain's response by way of intuitive reaction to a chemical imbalance has the desired effect. However, when the imbalances become too severe, or if something interferes with the brain's natural ability to regulate chemical production and release, we may end up with imbalance, disease, or illness. This is why it is so important to assist and influence our own brain chemistry with the proper exercise, nutrients, and sleep. In addition, specific movements and specific nutrients affect specific neurotransmitters. For example, balance exercises and methodical movements stimulate more of the calming chemicals, such as acetylcholine and serotonin, which slow the heart rate; on the other hand, kickboxing could stimulate more of the energy chemicals, such as dopamine and norepinephrine (noradrenaline), which increase the heart rate.

We will also look at many other things that have positive effects on the brain's chemistry, such as positive thinking, scents, music, gratitude, forgiveness, prayer, and meditation. The next chapter will provide more detailed information on specific neurotransmitters and hormones and how they affect our everyday lives. Before we move on, let's overview what we talked about earlier. Continuing our tour of the brain, let's look at the autonomic nervous system, the fight-or-flight mechanism, and the stress response. Here we will get a bit deeper and break down the responsibilities of each system. To make it easier to remember, we will use *warming* when referring to the sympathetic system and *cooling* when referring to the parasympathetic system.

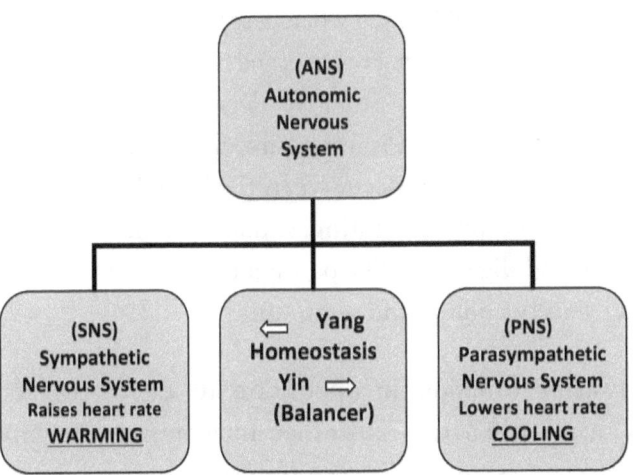

The *autonomic nervous system* (ANS) is responsible for regulation of internal organs, glands, and systems that, for the most part, we cannot control. This system is under the control of the subconscious but occurs unconsciously.

The autonomic nervous system regulates heart rate, respiratory rate, pupillary response, urination, and sexual arousal. The autonomic nervous system is further divided into two systems: the *sympathetic nervous system* (SNS) and the *parasympathetic nervous system* (PNS).[13]

I will use the word *warming* when I describe the *sympathetic nervous system* because its responsibilities are assertive and protective, increasing the heart rate. It is our fight-or-flight mechanism, getting us ready for action: increasing the heart rate, blood pressure, and blood flow, preparing us for action. The sympathetic nervous system is driven and dominated by dopamine and epinephrine (adrenaline).

---

13    Satterfield, Mind-Body Medicine, www.thegreatcourses.com.

The word *cooling* will be used when describing the *parasympathetic nervous system* because it is concerned with saving energy. The PNS is recuperative and restorative, decreasing the heart rate. To be more specific the PNS is responsible for stimulation of the *rest and digest* activities that occur when the body is at rest, calming us down—especially after eating, sexual arousal, salivation, tears, urination, and digestion. The parasympathetic nervous system is driven by acetylcholine and serotonin.

The systems function in opposition to each other but are complimentary in nature rather than antagonistic. The important thing to know is, *the PNS lowers the heart rate* (cooling) and the *SNS raises the heart rate* (warming). Maintaining a healthy balance between the two is necessary for emotional stability and physical health.

## Stress Response = Fight-or-Flight or Fright/Freeze

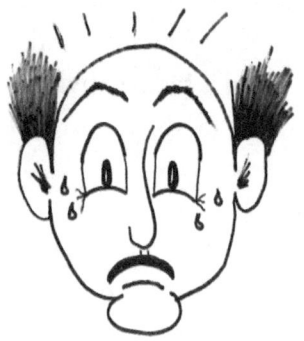

The *fight-or-flight response* is a physiological response to a perceived harmful event, attack, or threat to survival. The primary mechanism responsible for the fight-or-flight is the autonomic nervous system, and it acts, for the most part, out of our conscious control.

The stress response is activated in a number of ways, such as fear of danger, an accident, a traumatic event, an argument or disagreement, traffic, or any stressful event. To make matters even worse, thoughts (memory) of any of the situations mentioned also trigger the stress response.

The fight-or-flight mechanism works well when it goes through the full cycle, which is fear input, reaction/response, and resolution. Unfortunately, many of today's stressors do not allow us to complete the cycle. Most modern stressors are not attacks but more of challenges. If we look at the stress as an attack, so does the brain, and it will act accordingly.[14]

Below is a list of different activities: those on the *warming* side increase the heart rate and those on the *cooling* side decrease the heart rate. The examples below are a wide variety of activities and behaviors. By looking at this list, you may see which system is more active in your daily activities. These are just a few examples, but it should help you understand how we may lack balance in this system. Just keep in mind, if you are activating the system that raises your heart rate more often than not, you may be stressed out and not know it.

---

[14]  Satterfield, Mind-Body Medicine, www.thegreatcourses.com

## WARMING

### SNS
Raises Heart Rate
Raises Blood Pressure

Raises Respiratory Rate

Decreases Digestion

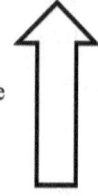

## COOLING

### PNS
Lowers Heart Rate
Lowers Blood Pressure
Lowers Respiratory Rate
Increases Digestion

### Activities/Behavior

| Warming (MonkeyBrain) | Cooling |
|---|---|
| Rushing/running late | Being prepared/ time efficient |
| Worrying about finances | Receiving a bonus or a gift |

| | |
|---|---|
| Loud noises or hard music | Sounds of nature or soft rhythmic music |
| Blaming or complaining | Praising or complimenting others |
| Doubt or pessimism | Trust or optimism |
| Insecurity/ Psychological fear | Feeling secure/ having faith |
| Re-living stress, fear or drama | Reframing negative thoughts |
| Arguments or disagreements | Communicating to solve problems |
| Traffic or waiting in long lines | Getting a front row parking spot |
| Stressful events | 10 deep diaphragmatic breaths |
| Real danger/fear (Fight-or-flight) | Removing yourself from danger |
| Anger and Pain | Forgiveness and empathy |
| Spinning/ kick boxing/power lifting | Yoga / Tai-Chi/Meditation |
| Resentment/Hate | Forgiveness /Love |
| Control | Acceptance |

Take a personal inventory of this list. Look at your daily activities. How often are you turning yourself up and how often are you turning yourself down? If you recognize an imbalance, take action to help bring yourself back to balance. Remember, what goes up must also come down.

Now let's look at the chemicals that correspond with the behavior and emotion. Although there are as many as fifty of these chemicals interacting with the brain and the body, the following are the main players. The specific actions and responsibilities of each chemical will follow in chapter 3.

| SNS – Raises heart rate | PNS – Lowers heart rate |
|---|---|
| Fight-or-flight | Rest and digest |
| Dopamine | Acetylcholine |

| Epinephrine (adrenalin) | Serotonin |
|---|---|
| Norepinephrine (noradranilin)) | Endorphins |
| Cortisol | GABA |
| DMT | Melatonin |
| | Vasopressin |
| | Oxytocin |
| | |

The most common cause of deficiency of cooling chemicals is feeling unsafe in your environment. Chronic worrying can be an hourly event for most who are deficient in cooling chemicals. This not only drains serotonin but also increases stress hormones, causing irritability, restlessness, and anxiety.

We will look at ways in which to improve the functions of these systems in chapter 4, but for now, let us look at the process known as *neuronal activity* or *neurotransmission*. Here we will review the specifics of each chemical.

# Chapter 3

# Neurotransmitters and Hormones

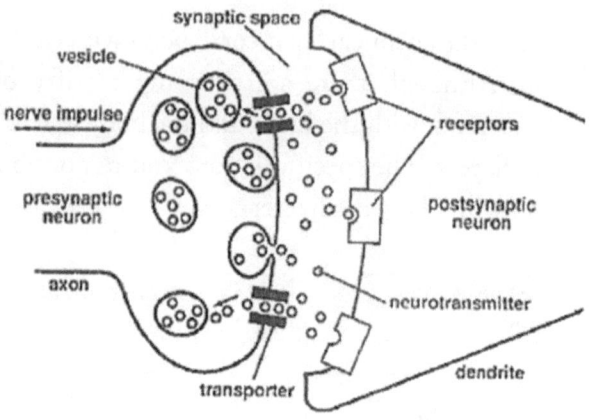

*Neurotransmission is the communication
highway from the brain to the body
~ Unknown*

One of the mysteries of brain science is how *neuronal activity* dictates behavior and even consciousness.[15] Neuronal activity is the brain's intricate balance of *neurotransmitters*. It is what determines how we feel. We are essentially the bodily manifestations of our neurotransmitters. Neurotransmitters run through the brain, directly to the central nervous system. Each transmitter has only one receptor that it can accept. The communication between the two plays some of the most active and significant roles in almost every function that a human body performs. These roles include: contracting muscles, relaying information, feeling excitement,

---

[15]     Wang, The Neuroscience of Everyday Life, www.thegreatcourses.com

feeling hunger or sleep, and feeling pain. All of these are a result of neuronal activity. Just imagine life without emotion or with out-of-control emotions. If one piece of this chemical puzzle is missing or damaged, the balance is compromised. There is a chemical reaction to everything that we do or do not do. For example, if you are walking down the street and you find a $100 bill or run into an old friend, your brain instantly releases a tiny bit of dopamine and serotonin, among other neurotransmitters, that makes you feel alert, happy, and even gives you a little boost of energy.

On the other hand, we can deplete our brain's chemicals and throw the brain's chemistry out of balance a number of ways. We could miss a good friend's birthday or be late for a meeting at work. Fear and guilt can make us feel bad about ourselves, depleting good feeling chemicals, turning our mood gloomy, and causing us to withdraw even more. This imbalance can lead to further feelings of doubt, insecurity, and confusion, causing a deeper imbalance.

When we stimulate multiple good feeling neurotransmitters, it makes us feel good. Enough of the good feeling neurotransmitters makes us feel energized and content, while a deficiency could leave us tired and unmotivated.

The good news is that we can influence neuronal activity with the proper nutrients and by our actions (sufficient sleep, proper movement, balanced nutrition, and forward thinking). In other words, we can influence the way that we feel by influencing the stimulation of specific neurotransmitters through various nutrients and actions. If you balance your brain chemistry, you can balance your emotions. Understanding which neurotransmitters are responsible for the way we feel can help us take the necessary action by way of activity, nutrition, environment, or attitude.

Although there are as many as fifty neurotransmitters, here we will focus on those that have been most studied. Below you will find a list of the main players and their specific responsibilities, as well as the feelings/emotions that they convey to the body. Since these chemicals determine how we think, speak, and act, understanding the communication between the chemicals and the messages that each convey to the body can assist us in influencing the balance. This gives us the opportunity to optimize our brain function and overall well-being.

- *Acetylcholine:* Cooling (PNS) is the "brainy" neurotransmitter, improving mental alertness and memory. It is the most abundant neurotransmitter in the body and is the primary neurotransmitter between neurons and muscles (neuromuscular feedback). It is the main driver for the parasympathetic nervous system, pulling other neurotransmitters to lower the heart rate. Acetylcholine is needed for learning and concentration. Deficiency can lead to memory loss, mood disorders, and possibly Alzheimer's disease. It helps the body perform a variety of construction work functions, such as neuronal connections (helping other neurotransmitters by making their connection stronger).
- *Epinephrine* (also known as *adrenaline)*: Warming (SNS) is the "motivator," stimulating you and helping you respond to stress.

    Adrenaline is associated with motivation, drive, energy, stimulation, and the stress response. It is also classified as a hormone. The adrenal glands are the core of the endocrine system's stress response. Two of their most important hormones are adrenaline and cortisol; they are responsible for the fight-or-flight response that controls how we deal with stress. When adrenaline is stimulated too often, it can create chronic stress patterns, thereby creating a biological change in the brain that allows for the constant release of cortisol and other harmful chemicals. In other words, the brain stays in a constant stress cycle with no end until the root of the stress is addressed.

- *Cortisol*: Warming (SNS) is a hormone produced by the adrenal cortex in response to stress. The fight-or-flight hormones are adrenaline or cortisol, which speed up the heart rate and create a heightened alert state to prepare the body for the stress: fight, flight, or even fright. However, the primary function of cortisol is to increase blood sugar levels as it aids in fat, carbohydrate, and protein metabolism. Cortisol plays a very important role in the stress response, cardiovascular health, and immune system. The proper amount of cortisol is crucial to the balance of these systems. Over- or underproduction of cortisol due to stress and overeating sugars and starches will disrupt the balance and can eventually cause illness and possibly diseases, such as diabetes, heart disease, and stroke.

- *Norepinephrine* (also known as *noradrenaline*): Warming (SNS) is similar to epinephrine (adrenaline) in regards to the brain's stress response. However, unlike epinephrine, norepinephrine is a positive stress response that is stimulated during sex, love, and exercise. Noradrenalin can also be activated with music, dancing, and extreme fun.

- *Dopamine:* Warming (SNS) dopamine is the neurotransmitter that has significance in many behaviors. Dopamine is made in a section of the brain called the *basil ganglia* that is implicated in movement. It is important in executive function, in reward, and in the regulation of movement. It is the feel-good neurotransmitter that make us feel energized and in control. Dopamine is associated with pleasure, motivation, alertness, concentration, and euphoria. In addition, both dopamine and noradrenaline are made from the amino acid tyrosine. Dopamine, however, seems to be the primary neurotransmitter of reward. Adequate levels of dopamine allow us to focus, to complete a task, to feel motivated, and to have energy. Low levels are associated with depression, lack of concentration, poor motivation, and difficulty initiating or completing tasks.

- *Endorphins*: Cooling (PNS) promote bliss, giving the sense of euphoria. Endorphins are associated with pleasure, orgasm, euphoria, and pain relief. Runners call endorphins the *runners high*. Endorphins are the brain's natural opiates. Low levels of endorphins are associated with mental and physical pain, addiction, and risk-taking behavior: the more reason to exercise regularly.

- *GABA (gamma-aminobutryic acid):* Cooling (PNS) is the "cool" neurotransmitter, relaxing you and calming you down after stress. GABA is one of the most researched neurotransmitters and plays an important role in relaxation, sedation, and sleep. Adequate levels of GABA lead to emotional tranquility, while low levels are associated with anxiety, tension, and insomnia. GABA is an amino acid that acts as an inhibitory neurotransmitter. Inhibitory neurotransmitters decrease the electrochemical activity of neurons.

- *Serotonin*: Cooling (PNS) is the "happy" neurotransmitter, improving our mood and satisfaction. Serotonin is associated with sleep patterns, dreams, and visions. It influences many physiological functions, including blood pressure, digestion, body temperature, and pain sensations. Adequate levels provide emotional and social stability, while low levels are associated with depression, anxiety, carbohydrate cravings; sleep disturbances, increased sensitivity to pain, obsessive thinking, and alcohol and drug abuse.

- *Oxytocin:* Cooling (PNS) is known to some as the "moral molecule." Oxytocin is both a hormone and a neurotransmitter. It is released during childbirth, breast feeding, and pair and maternal bonding. In addition, recent studies have shown additional activities that stimulate oxytocin are touch, orgasm, helping others (acts of service), being compassionate, gratitude, sharing, mercy, trusting others, prayer, and meditation. Oxytocin has the ability to inhibit the amygdala, thereby blocking the release of cortisol, giving it the name "anti-stress hormone." My personal opinion is that oxytocin is the antagonist to cortisol and is required to help regulate stress. If there is such a thing as the God molecule, oxytocin is it!

- *Vasopressin*: Cooling (PNS) is very similar to oxytocin in function; however, men seem to have more vasopressin than women. Women seem to have much more stimulation of oxytocin than men. The action potential in both is alike, with some slight differences. Vasopressin also has the ability to inhibit the release of stress hormones, placing this hormone in the stress-reducing category.

- *Melatonin*: Cooling (PNS) it regulates your inner clock for day and night, and helps with sleep. Melatonin also acts as an anti- depressant with anti-aging properties. However, its main role seems to be keeping you in sync with the rhythms of nature. It harmonizes brain function with day and night.

- *DHEA:* Cooling (PNS) a hormone believed by some to be an effective marker of a person's biological age. Some data suggest that low DHEA levels are inversely related to the likelihood of acquiring age-related conditions, such as cardiovascular disease, diabetes, and cancer.

- *DMT (dimethyltryptamine)*: Cooling (PNS) helps you see the big picture. It is associated with peak experiences and major insights. DMT is thought to be produced in the pineal gland, along with serotonin and melatonin. It is thought to be released at birth, facilitating an infant's transition from womb to world. It is also released at death.

- *Glutamate*: Warming (SNS) has critical roles in learning and memory. However an excess of glutamate induces *excitotoxicity*, a route by which neurons are damaged. To better explain this: neurotransmitters classified as excitatory or inhibitory are based on their effects on postsynaptic neuron membranes. A neurotransmitter can be called *excitatory* if activation of the receptor promotes action potential generation. A neurotransmitter can be called *inhibitory* if the activation of the receptor depresses action potential generation. Glutamate is classified as excitatory.

Neurotransmission is the way that neurons communicate. The electrical synapses are the direct connections between neurons; however, the most common way of communication is chemical communication using neurotransmitters. In order to influence the way that we feel, we must influence the chemistry of the brain in one direction or another. And we do this through our thoughts, actions, reactions, nutrients, and environment. The chapter on neurotransmitters is provided as a reference guide.

We are each unique and different in our brain chemistry makeup, and understanding the responsibilities of each chemical can help us maintain our unique balance. This chapter can be used as a reference when designing your exercise program, meal plan, and supplementation, if needed. But for now, let us move on to chapter 4, the cause and effects of stress and fear.

# CHAPTER 4

# Stress and Fear

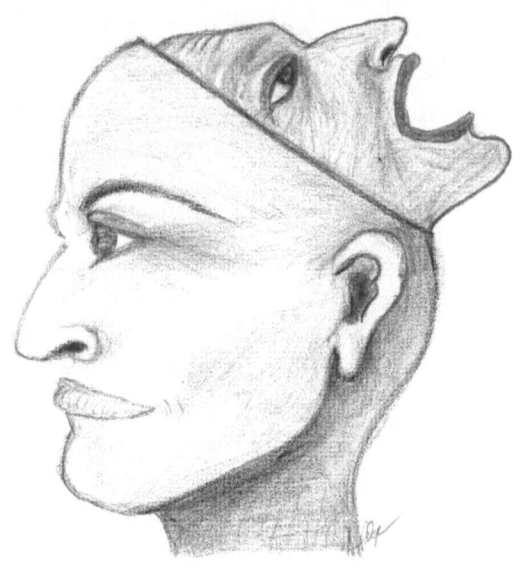

*Anxiety is the feeling that one has to do something or
the feeling of not having finished something.*
*~ Unknown*

I felt compelled to research the origins of stress and fear for two reasons. First, stress and fear seem to come up in almost every conversation, whether with my clients, family, or friends. Second, it fuels the emergence of the MonkeyBrain, which we do not want to happen.

The fight-or-flight stress response has the following effect on the physical body: it increases breathing and the heart rate, it elevates blood pressure, and it raises blood-sugar levels. The stress response prepares the body for self-defense or escape, hence the name fight-or-flight. Fright can also trigger a stress response.[16] This mechanism worked fine when we were running from predators during the beginning of human existence. Now, however, as much as we would like to, we cannot run from annoying neighbors, a stalled car, or a bitter boss. Unlike our ancestors, we have no way of burning off this excess energy. It is this excess energy that keeps us in a stress mode. As a matter of fact, animals in the wild go through a series of movements that disperse the energy and complete the stress cycle right away. Once an animal has escaped from whatever was causing their stress, they stomp their legs up and down until they have released the stressful energy. Humans usually do not release stressful energy, so the stress cycle for most of us living in modern society does not have a beginning and an end.

For example, if we encounter a dangerous situation in real time, the fight-or-flight mechanism is activated and the chemicals are stimulated to make us very alert and aware of our surroundings. Once the situation has improved or we remove ourselves from the danger, different chemicals are then stimulated that make us feel calm and at ease. This is the complete cycle. However, in today's society, we have many stressors, such as work, traffic, running late, and many modern life experiences that also trigger the stress response. These stressors stimulate chemicals and hormones, such as epinephrine (adrenaline) and cortisol. If the stress is prolonged, it will have negative effects on our health as a whole. Remember, one of the primary functions of cortisol is to balance blood-sugar levels. Unfortunately, overproduction will disrupt that balance, which can then lead to diabetes, circulatory issues, and additional storage of body fat in the belly region. Added to the physical

---

[16]    Satterfield, Mind-Body Medicine, www.thegreatcourses.com

burden, we store mental images of stressful and traumatic events for many years. These events can pop up in our memories at any time. The mere thought of these events can trigger the same chemical reaction exactly as if the event were occurring again in real time. Most of our stress is only in our head. Most stresses are not disasters. However, thinking they are can overwhelm us. The problem doesn't have to be real or present; it can be past or future. To make things even worse, persistent stress in real time or in one's head can have negative and unhealthy effects on the growth of neurons. Remember, neurons transport chemical messengers (neurotransmitters).

Psychological stress and fear includes: doubt, anger, jealousy, resentment, and even embarrassment. Most of these emotions stem from mismanaged negative thoughts of fear. For example, a person who is worried about an upcoming exam or a big project at work begins to feel restless and have sweaty palms, dry mouth, or a queasy stomach. These are all stress warnings triggered by the stress response. The stress begins with fear. Examples would be: fear of failure, fear of what others will say, or fear of being fired. It is compulsive thinking and most of it is repetitive and pointless.

Stress that is caused by thoughts does not always go through the *stress cycle* of *fear input, reaction, and resolution.* A pattern of psychological fear or stress seems to continuously re-loop while prolonging the body's stress response and creating a chronic release of adrenaline and cortisol. This is also known as *chronic anxiety.*

Epinephrine (adrenaline) is significantly important because it stimulates our drive and motivation. Also, over time, the brain becomes addicted to adrenalin. Many experiences stimulate adrenaline. If stress has been your primary stimulator, when the stress goes away and your brain begins to withdraw from the adrenaline, it will seek even more stress to gain relief. Remember, the MonkeyBrain will be looking for a way to create more drama in your life, creating an increase in the need for more and more adrenaline.

Real life is impossible without stress. We cannot completely avoid it. There are many levels of stress and fear. Each of us has our stress makers that trigger the stress response. We do need a certain amount of stress to stimulate the mind and the body, but unfortunately, life in the modern world brings with it stresses that we can live without, specifically anxiety.

Anxiety is just chronic stress. Over time, fear and stress patterns become chronic, and the brain may consolidate the connection into another region of the brain where it is not as noticeable to us when it is happening. This is when it becomes chronic anxiety! This can play a major role on the brain and body's balance. Imbalance is what can cause negative health issues, and it all begins with the imbalance of neurotransmitters (the chemicals that communicate from neuron to neuron). There are also stressors that are out of our control, such as pollution in our air, water, and food supply. These pollutants all create some chaos and stress for the brain and body but can be managed with balanced nutrients, sleep, and proper exercise.

So what does stress do to the health of our brain and body? Stress triggers a chemical response that disrupts the chemical make-up in our brain. Remember, neurotransmitters affect the brain, and hormones affect the body. There is an internal biological and chemical balance that the brain and body want to maintain. Humans and most animals are equipped with a very sophisticated mechanism set up to seek that balance. As mentioned earlier, *homeostasis* is the body's balancing mechanism that regulates serotonin and dopamine, the yin and the yang of the human body.

Homeostasis is part of the autonomic nervous system, which includes the sympathetic and parasympathetic nervous systems. We looked at this system in Chapter 2. It is the regulating system of the brain doing its best to maintain a positive balance. Prolonged stress disrupts the chemical makeup and biological system, eventually causing cell damage, illness, and disease. Therefore, reducing stress is a sure way to improve our brain, body, and mind. Physical exercise is one of the most efficient ways to do this.

Exercise does this by improving the balance of your brain's chemistry. It also improves your heart and lung function, improves metabolism, reduces body fat, and increases lean body mass. This helps you deal better with stress.

Stress of any kind creates a toxic chemical byproduct such as free radicals. Free radicals damage living tissue and cause healthy cells to oxidize and become unhealthy chaotic cells. Think of it this way: when fruits or vegetables are left out for a length of time, they will oxidize and rot. Free radicals basically do the same thing to the human cell. This is why antioxidants can help combat free radical damage to human cells. Antioxidants that are found in most fruits and vegetables help mop up the free radical cells, which are oxidizing, blocking further damage to healthy cells. Eating foods that are rich in antioxidants can help to reduce stress.

Although exercise is good for reducing stress, it can cause free radical damage and create inflammation at the same time. This damage can be detoxified with proper rest, nutrients, and antioxidants.

Dr. Hans Seelye, Nobel Prize winner and the father of stress research proposed that the fight-or-flight stress response has three stages. Seelye described it as *General Adaptation Syndrome* or GAS. The stages are alarm, adaptation, and finally exhaustion. His model is useful in helping to see where one is in the stress cycle and what to do about it.

## *Three stages of stress: alarm, adaptation, and exhaustion.*

The first stage of stress is the *alarm stage*. During this stage, the brain signals specific glands to produce stress hormones to come to the rescue. Although there are as many as forty such hormones, the most important, in regards to the stress response, are adrenaline, cortisol, and dehydroepiandrosterone (DHEA). At the moment that we are alarmed, the adrenaline effect kicks in and then slowly begins to diminish, while the cortisol keeps on coming. Both adrenaline and cortisol boost your blood sugar. The adrenals also release the hormone DHEA, which helps maintain energy and resistance to stress.

As a result of this rapid release of these chemicals, our body is supplied with more oxygen and sugar, allowing more blood to the brain and muscles. This additional energy makes us very alert and prepares the brain, the muscles, and the organs for fight-or-flight. The rapid increase in chemicals, in fact, gives us a bit of a high. This is precisely why we can create stress in our lives just to experience this stimulation. It may be stress, but it's also a high for the brain. The MonkeyBrain loves stress.

The *adaptation stage* is when the body needs to continue its defense mechanism beyond the fight-or-flight response. As we enter the adaptation stage, cortisol and DHEA have a reciprocal relationship. The cortisol levels go up, and DHEA levels drop.

This is when we start to feel the effects of long-term stress, with increasing anxiety, fatigue, and mood swings.

The *exhaustion stage* is when we become stuck in the stress response. It becomes chronic. The exhaustion phase is dangerous because we can no longer produce the necessary cortisol to respond to stress, and our DHEA levels drop. Also we deplete the vitamins C, Bs, and essential minerals, such as magnesium. This drains us of energy and motivation.[17]

Short-term stress (adaptation stage) comes at a high cost and does the following:

- *Suppresses the immune system, increasing risk of infections*
- *Slows digestion*
- *Slows down metabolism*
- *Increases heart rate and release of cortisol*

In the long-term, (exhaustion stage), stress will do the following:

- *Increases risk of developing high blood pressure, diabetes, heart disease, and digestive problems.*
- *Depletes the body of vitamins, especially vitamin C*
- *Leads to weight gain*
- *Promotes rapid aging*

Short and long-term stress may cause the following symptoms:

- *Vague aches and pains*
- *Muscle tension*
- *Heart burn*

---

[17]    Selye, Birth of Stress, info@stress.org.

- *Dry mouth*
- *Fatigue*
- *Insomnia*
- *Sugar cravings*
- *Racing heart rate*
- *Racing thoughts*
- *Mood swings*
- *Recurring headaches*

What phase are you in? The question is not if the stress will come, it is how prepared are you to deal with it when the stress comes. It is less about the stressor and more about the coping skills. The following techniques can and should be used to help deal with stress in more productive ways:

1. *Breathe deeply*: When you start to feel tense, take ten deep breaths through your diaphragm, not just through your chest. Fill the belly first, and then the lungs, and allow the breath to be fully released. You can breathe through the discomfort. Deep breathing shifts the autonomic nervous system from the sympathetic nervous system (raises the heart rate) to the parasympathetic nervous system (lowers the heart rate), reducing the stress hormones and the stress.

2. *Adopt healthy eating habits*: We deal with stress more effectively when we are not lacking the proper nutrients. We will also feel better when our diet is balanced. Try to include foods high in fiber, such as beans, berries, and whole grains. Always include some source of protein, whether it is lean meats, tofu, eggs, or low fat dairy products. Also include polyunsaturated or monounsaturated fats, such as nuts, olives, sunflower seeds, or olive and canola oils. Drink a minimum of 32 oz. of water daily, and reduce

your intake of caffeine, alcohol, fried foods, salt, and sugar. More details in Part II.

3. *Practice effective time management*: You will be under less pressure if you prepare early, set goals, do time audits, and establish priorities with a list. A list preps the brain and reduces the thoughts of having forgotten to do something. This allows you to focus your attention on each thing as you are doing it. Remember, anxiety is the feeling of having to do something and the feeling of not having finished something. The list can help you avoid these feelings. Avoid overscheduling. You cannot manage time, but you can manage yourself. And remember, procrastination can cause stress and anxiety. Avoid procrastination at all cost.

4. *Accept change*: Change is an important part of life. Learn to adapt to detours. Experience the fullness of the detour as a new experience with valuable lessons. Accept the fact that your job, relationships, and life in general will produce changes to which you must adjust. Some of the most drastic changes in my life have been among the most important life lessons. Sometimes the detours are just signs to slow down, pay attention, be in the moment, and enjoy life as it comes: good, bad, or indifferent. Embrace all experiences at the moment. Change can be a very good thing.

5. *Keep a sense of humor*: Look for the humor in every situation. Even a slight smile can stimulate the release of rewarding chemicals that can reduce stress. Fake it until you break it. Surround yourself with people and things that make you laugh out loud. Harness that energy and spread it to others.

6. *Get physical*: Participate in some form of regular physical activity. Exercise, play sports, dance, or wash your car.

Home projects such as cleaning house, gardening, mowing your lawn, or renovating projects do count. Just move! Consistent forward movement with a purpose also encourages forward thinking. It is movement of the body that stimulates positive rewarding chemicals in the brain that make us feel better. Purposeful motion, with devotion, creates balanced emotions. This is the magic potion.

7. *Patrol your thoughts*: Be aware of the voice in your head. If the thoughts are making you feel bad, shift the thought to memories that make you feel good. Remember, the brain can pull memory/thoughts without your consent, and those thoughts could be bad for your health. Beware! Direct your thoughts in the direction of your dreams and goals. Think of the solution to whatever problem you may be having.

8. *Write a daily to-do list*: First identify the projects that need to be completed. *Don't just think it; write it.* Break down large projects into smaller tasks. Write it down. Set reasonable deadlines and write the date. Schedule the tasks for when you are the most productive. Reward yourself for accomplishing each task by *scratching* each off once it has been completed. The brain sees accomplishment as a reward and will release more chemicals, such as dopamine and serotonin, which give you more motivation and enhance your mood. Take note: getting started is often the most difficult part. We can expend more energy avoiding the task than is needed to complete the task. The list will also help reduce stress by avoiding procrastination.

Any time a problem arises, always start to think of the best-case scenario. Thinking this way helps the brain/mind find the means to manifest those desires. If you find yourself reliving stressful or painful experiences in your head, shift the thought to the solution. You could also use music, funny movies, pets, nature, or just take a walk to shift the chemicals that help reduce stressful thoughts. It is up to us to choose the direction.

Life is often difficult and stressful. Try to keep your life in balance. Your job, family, friends, education, helping others, fun, and leisure time are all important. If you ignore one completely to concentrate on another, you are at risk of upsetting the balance, which allows you to handle stress as it comes your way. We cannot avoid stress; we can only mange it. Take an inventory of the things that you are trying to balance and modify your time accordingly.

The following questionnaire can help you recognize some of the signs and see where you fit on the stress continuum. In the following questionnaire, mark *yes* if the question applies more than half of the time. Score 1 point for each *yes* answer.

## How Stressed Are You?

- Do you have problems sleeping? \_\_\_\_
- Do you lack interest in sex? \_\_\_\_
- Do you have difficulty delegating? \_\_\_\_
- Do you often have dry mouth and sweaty palms? \_\_\_\_
- Do you eat quickly? \_\_\_\_
- Do you take on too much? \_\_\_\_
- Do you have difficulty relaxing? \_\_\_\_
- Are you often irritable? \_\_\_\_
- Are you unable to shut off your mind? \_\_\_\_
- Do you find it hard to relate to other people? \_\_\_\_
- Are you impatient with others? \_\_\_\_

- Do you worry about the little events of the day? _____
- Do you smoke or drink excessively? _____
- Are you overly competitive? _____

*Scoring:*

1-5: You are basically at a normal stress level. You could use some of the techniques mentioned earlier to calm down as the challenges arise.

6-10: You are quite stressed. Pay attention to these warning signs and use as many of the stress-reducing techniques as it takes to reduce your stress level.

11-14: You are in a dangerous stress stage. It is time to clean up your act before there are serious health consequences. You will need to use exercise, nutrition, and sleep to bring your stress level down. Use any of the stress-reducing techniques provided in *MonkeyBrain* on a regular basis to help manage your stress levels, including supplements if needed. [18]

Remember, the techniques provided for reducing stress only work when you use them on a regular basis. It is much easier to deal with stress if the brain and the body have been conditioned to deal with these neurological and physiological challenges. Proper exercise, balanced nutrition, and sufficient sleep are most important for reducing stress levels. These three things strengthen and regulate the body's natural defense mechanisms. All of the other techniques are additional tools for managing and reducing stress as it comes.

---

[18]   Seyle, Birth of Stress, Info@stress.org.

Before we move on to the practical work, we need to look at additional resources for coping. This would be considered your social support group. Most of us have different people (resources) in our lives that help us through stressful situations. Here are the different types of support:

- Emotional support
- Informational/advice support
- Financial support
- Intimacy/trust support

Let's begin with emotional support. This is a person who would help you feel better emotionally or help you feel better about the stressful situation. This person will give you comfort.

Informational/advice support is that person or connection that can give you advice. This person could help you get the right information that you need to clear up the problem. This would be that resourceful person who can help you find the solution to the problem. It could be a friend, your boss, or information that you received from the web.

Next would be financial support. This is the person who you know has the financial resources to help you in a time of need. The financial aid will help relieve the stress.

At last, we have intimacy and trust support. This would be the person who you trust the most. This is the person who knows you best and will support you through thick and thin. This can include spiritual support.

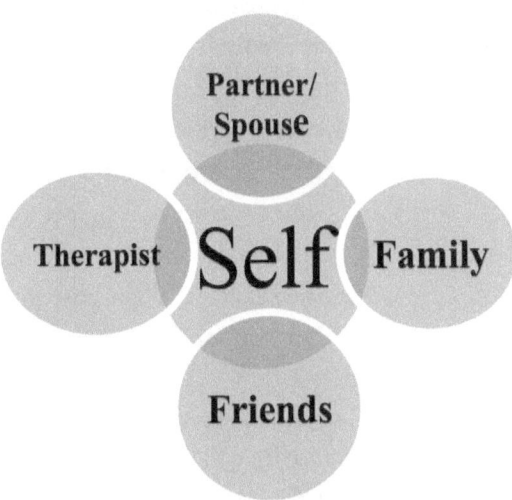

Now imagine yourself in the middle circle, and your resources are spouse or partner, family, friends, and maybe a therapist or support group. Write down the names of the people in each support circle. Then apply the appropriate support with that person. Let's look at an example:

*Social Support Group*

1. Spouse/partner
2. Family member
3. Friends
4. Therapist/support group
5. Pets

Here you can see five different areas of support, each supplying you with different resources. For example, you could get advice and emotional support from your therapist, but don't expect much financial aid. Or you may turn to your family members for emotional and intimacy support, but they may not have the resources to help you with financial stress. It all depends on what type of stress you are going through and what type of support would be best for that situation. If you are lucky, you may have one or two people in your support group that could provide you with any of the resources that you need. If it is emotional support that you need, spending some time with your pet could be the perfect resource to shift your mood. Take an inventory of your support group. First, write their names. Then next to each name, write down in which way they support you. For example:

- Spouse/Partner: a.) Financial support, b.) Intimacy/ trust support, c.) Informative support
- Family: a.) Intimacy/trust support, b.) Emotional support
- Friends: a.) Informative support/advice
- Pets: a.) Emotional support

Here you can see how each person in this support group could provide different resources.[19] When you know what support each person can give you, you can then go straight to the resource the first time around. No more wasting time hoping your pet will give you advice or expecting to get financial aid from your therapist. Remember, the right resource can help you reduce your stress much sooner. Now let's look at ways in which to improve brain function.

---

[19] Satterfield, Mind-Body Medicine, www.thegreatcourses.com.

# CHAPTER 5

# Conditioning the Brain

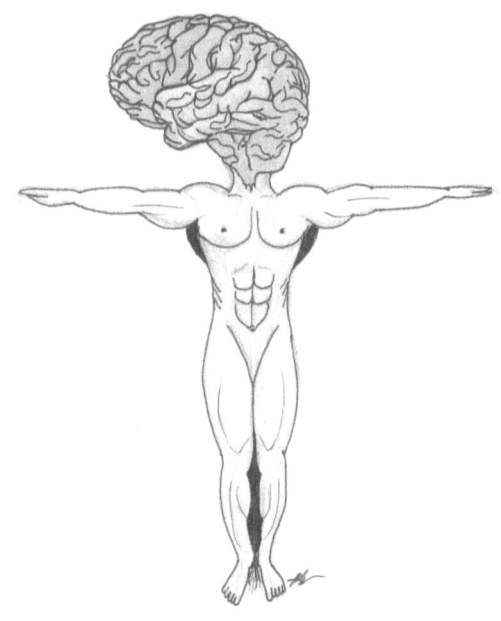

*If you don't use it, you lose it.*
*~Unknown*

Can we increase the power of our brain?

It turns out that we can increase the power of our brain at any time in life. Dr. Richard Restak, Professor of Medicine and Health Sciences at George Washington University, teaches that we can increase the power of our brain through our own efforts and actions. He goes on to say that culture, not biology, is now the greatest influence in brain development because the brain has plasticity, and plasticity is the brain's ability to change in response to experience. This means we can learn, develop, and improve brain function at any age. Even though sensory and social depravation early in life can lead to decreased intelligence, poor emotional health, and inability to adapt, the brain is dependent on our experiences and continues to evolve and develop throughout our lives. Dependence on the richness of environmental stimulation is not limited to early development. Our activities and thoughts are modifying our brains at every moment, regardless of age.

Dr. Restek also believes balanced diet, exercise, and sleep are critical for optimal brain functioning. Research has shown that exercise brings about positive changes in the brain function of children and adults. Also, more sleep and power naps have been shown to enhance memory consolidation and cognitive performance.[20]

He goes on to say, the overreliance on electronic information aids has resulted in disuse atrophy of our memory powers. We will review examples for improving our mental abilities in the next section. This loss of our ability to remember things can be overcome by deliberate effort and actions to improve memory. [21]Specifics are provided in the next section on brain training. The following examples are exercises to improve the power of our brains, making us better!

---

[20]   Restak, Optimizing Brain Fitness, www.thegreatcourses.com
[21]   Restak, Optimizing Brain Fitness, www.thegreatcourses.com

## Brain Training

The brain is an extraordinary organ, but it requires continued maintenance. In other words, if we don't use it, we lose it.

The following examples are brain-training exercises:

- Mental exercises, such as jigsaw puzzles, Sudoku, cryptograms, crossword puzzles, word division, and fill-in puzzles
- Card games, such as bridge, poker, and solitaire
- Learning new information of any kind
- Learning new skills, such as cooking, crochet, a new sport, or a musical instrument
- Computer games/memory games, such as Lumosity
- Writing/journaling
- Meditation

All of these activities improve the functions and processes of the brain, including memory and improved ability in focus and attention. Since we are all unique in the way we learn, this training is best left up to you. Choose any of the recommended brain training activities. Make a commitment (twenty minutes per day, three times per week), set a schedule to do the work, and document your participation in the twenty-one-day challenge, (located at the end of Part III).

Try something different each week. The twenty-one-day journal should be used to help you track your progress. For those of you who prefer something different every day, *MonkeyBrain* provides a sample seven-day quick-start program in the next section. Log your brain-training activity and duration of that session. In addition use the emotional checklist to document your feelings, mood, energy level, and overall attitude. This will allow you to see what activities help you feel and think better.

Now let us review what we have learned so far about the brain, its functions, and its chemistry. First, the three most important components for optimal brain function are: balanced diet, proper exercise, and sufficient sleep.

We also know that stress and fear fuel the MonkeyBrain and create more anxiety. Remember, the MonkeyBrain is a way of thinking that can be changed at any time.

Neurotransmitters and hormones are the chemicals that communicate and convey information from the brain to the body, and vice versa. These chemicals work individually or with one another, while some have the ability to activate each other. We know that all of these chemicals determine how we feel: good, bad, or indifferent. Also remember that emotional memory can stimulate the same chemicals as the original event, good or bad.

It is your thoughts that are creating the threat. But you can reframe your thoughts or use distraction through movement. And this can lead to resolving the stress. These are just two behavior modifications that enable the complete cycle, which is fear input, reaction/response, and resolution. Refer back to Chapter 4 for more stress-reducing techniques.

Now that we know better, we can do better. With additional stressors in today's world, we must introduce more stress-reducing techniques. These additional tools help develop new feedback systems for reducing stress hormones. When our brain chemistry becomes unbalanced, we must take the necessary action to return to balance. We can use movement, nutrition, sleep, or change of environment.

We also know that humans have two opposing hormone responses to stimuli. The first is the fight-or-flight hormones, known as dopamine, epinephrine aka/adrenaline, and cortisol, which speed up the heart rate and create a hyper-alert state of mind.

The other hormone responses are acetylcholine, serotonin, GABA, and oxytocin, which balance the fight-or-flight response and have the opposite effect by slowing the heart rate down. Maintaining this balance is necessary for optimum brain function, emotional stability, and overall health.

We also know that we can enhance brain function by learning new information of any kind. For example, look up a new word in the dictionary and its definition; write it, read it, and memorize it. This works several areas of memory, and although it is usually not long-term, it exercises the functions of short-term memory. This type of brain training can end those days of misplacing your keys or wallet, or not remembering if you closed the garage door.

*Writing a list* can also help you remember. Writing a list of the things that you have to accomplish for that day allows the brain to focus on other things instead of obsessing about what has to be done or what has not been done. It is important that you scratch off each task and give yourself credit for completing that task. No matter how small or large the task is, the brain will still take the win. This simple list has multiple benefits, such as helping you stay organized, consciously directing your day, and reducing stress by avoiding procrastination. More important, over time, doing a list every day can improve confidence and increase will power.

Another way to improve your brain is through acquiring new skills, such as learning a new sport, learning a new language, cooking a new recipe, or learning how to play a musical instrument.

The learning of any new skill will enhance brain function while stimulating good feeling chemicals. In addition, the data also indicates that computer games, word games, number games, and different types of puzzles improve brain function, memory, and ability to focus and concentrate. [22]

Brain training requires focus and attention, and is best done alone. There is no multitasking in brain training. It is all about focus and attention on the task in front of you. Remember, focus and attention improves learning and physical performance. In addition to brain training, it is also important to do work for the mind: mind training.

Mind training is very different. As a matter of fact, it is the opposite of brain training. The goal is to slow down, lower the heart rate, and relax the brain and body. More specifics on mind training will be provided in Part III.

We can now move on to the practical work of brain training. Determine which works best for you. Since we are all unique, it is best to try many different exercises, including the ones that you may not prefer. Similar to cross training the physical body by using different exercises, cross training the brain with different exercises conditions the brain in more ways, which provides better results. Below you will find a seven-day brain-training regimen. Practice each exercise for that day.

Seven-Day *Quick Start* Brain-Training Program

- Day One: Memory work. Look up a new word in the dictionary and memorize the word and the definition. Read it, write it, and memorize it. Log the time that it

---

[22] Restak, Optimizing Brain Fitness, www.thegreatcourses.com

took for you to complete the task in the twenty-one-day challenge. Just do one word and its definition for this day.

- Day Two: Play card games (poker, bridge, or solitaire). Play for twenty to thirty minutes.
- Day Three: Read. Read at least one chapter of any book or article that provides you with new information. Use a wide variety of topics: history, science, arts, health, sports, fashion, and biographies.
- Day Four: Meditate five to twenty minutes.
- Day Five: Use computer learning games, memory games, or video games—without violence, if possible. (Keep this training to a maximum of thirty minutes per day if there is violence involved.)
- Day Six: Write or journal for ten to twenty minutes. Write poems, stories, and intentions for life, a gratitude journal, or anything that stimulates your creativity or imagination.
- Day Seven: Begin to learn a new skill, such as:
  1. A new sport (golf, tennis, bowling, skiing, surfing, etc.)
  2. A musical instrument
  3. How to sew or crochet
  4. The mechanics of yoga or an aerobics step class
  5. A new language
  6. How to paint

Learning a new skill takes practice and committed action over time. You don't have to be perfect overnight. Give yourself some time to learn a new skill without judgment, and enjoy the process. I was able to draw the illustrations for this book because I've practiced the skill of drawing for many years. It isn't so much that I have extraordinary talent; it is more about the commitment to keep trying until I became better at it. In today's society, we expect instant gratification, which doesn't work when learning a craft or skill.

After following the exercises provided in the Quick Start, you can then choose your own. Cross train your brain by using different exercises. Remember to log your activity in the twenty-one-day journal.

Before we move on to the physical, let's review the three cornerstones to optimum brain function.

The first cornerstone is to meet the *nutritional needs* for the brain by providing the brain with balanced meals of protein, carbohydrates, and fats. The brain requires all nutrients to perform optimally, and any deficiency has the ability to affect physical and mental performance. These nutrients are the fuel for your brain and your body. Part II will provide more specifics on nutrition and natural supplements to help determine what works best for your goals and needs.

The second cornerstone is *sleep*. The proper amount of sleep and rest is very specific to each person. However, the brain and the physical body do require time to rebuild and recuperate. Most of that work is done during sleep and rest. Allow yourself six to eight hours of sleep every twenty-four hours, and use power naps whenever possible.

The third cornerstone is *regular exercise*.[23] Choose movement of your choice. Some is better than others, but all movement counts. More specifics on proper exercises will be provided in Part II.

Now we can move on to the physical body and ways to improve it.

---

23    Restak, Optimizing Brain Fitness, www.thegreatcourses.com.

# PART II

# *The Physical Body*

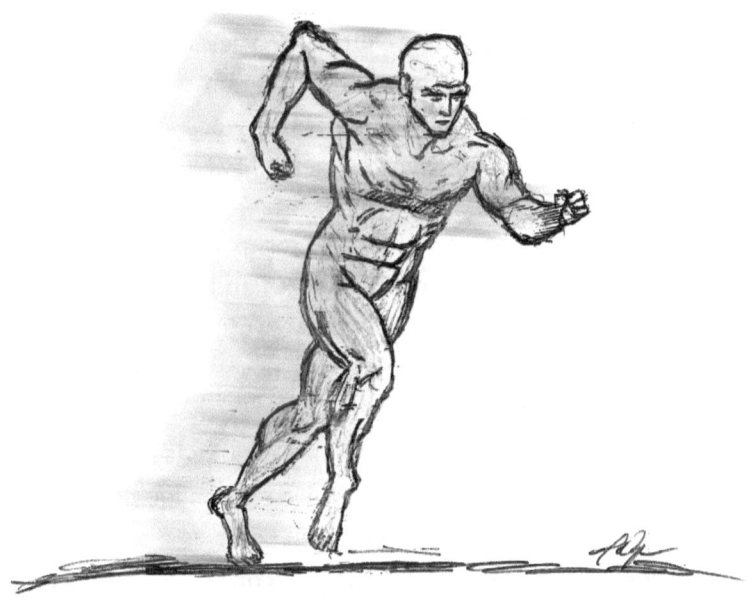

*No matter how slow you go, you are still
lapping everybody on the couch.*
~ Fitsugar

In Part I, we looked at some things that make us sick and some of the things that make us better. Here we will introduce the things that make us well. This chapter provides the needed framework for assisting you in developing a personalized program for exercise. But first, let us talk about the needs of the physical body. Optimum physical conditioning requires proper movement, balanced nutrition, and sufficient sleep. These three things are the cornerstones to optimum physical and mental performance and should be the foundation to any physical fitness conditioning program.

Part II will focus on assessing your fitness level and developing a personalized fitness program. This program will be designed to improve strength, muscular endurance, cardiovascular conditioning and develop balanced flexibility.

Since we know that sports and other forms of physical activity can serve as pathways to personal growth and development, the goal is to integrate the approach. First we know that physical exercise elevates mood and temporarily relieves feelings of stress and anxiety. In addition, exercise improves the cardiovascular system, metabolism, and cholesterol profile, builds muscle tissue, and burns body fat. It is a win/win however you look at it. More important, the potential for exercise to serve as a safe training ground for developing and changing behavior and emotional patterns is significant. The methods that will be provided for personal change rely on the fundamentals of fitness and active living.

Here is where the process begins. Through exercise alone, you will begin to improve your health, your brain function, and your awareness of the mind/body connection. Through practice and committed action over time, you will also begin to change behavior and emotional patterns, such as improving self-confidence and developing better self-reliance (coping skills) and stronger will power. The benefits of physical exercise can also increase your ability to focus and concentrate. In addition, exercise can allow you to create better social interactions. The nutritional component will be discussed in detail in chapter seven. But for now, let us take a brief look at the muscular system.

It is important to know how the muscular system works and how we can influence the balance of this system. Although physiology is a complex subject, here we will discuss the basic fundamentals that affect our everyday lives. For the purpose of easy understanding, I will keep this as simple as possible. A *skeletal muscle* is composed of groups of hairlike fibers that join into a *tendon* at each end. Each fiber is a cell in itself and can change length when nerve impulses stimulate it, as when we move our body.

The energy for the movement of working muscles comes from the oxygen and nutrients supplied to the cell by the heart, lungs, and blood vessels. This supply is fueled by the food and liquids that we ingest. The endurance of a muscle can be understood by its capacity to use energy in order to contract, to cause movement, and to prevent fatigue.

The energy to these cells is supplied by the foods we eat. The oxygen in our bloodstream is utilized within the muscle cell in a series of chemical reactions to form *adenosine triphosphate* (ATP). ATP is found in every cell of the body and is necessary for contracting muscles, performing other cell processes that require energy, and conducting nerve impulses. Once ATP is used up, it must be replenished by way of more food (nutrients) and oxygen. When the ATP is not restored in time, an ample supply of oxygen is not available in the muscles, therefore activating another mechanism to rebuild the ATP immediately. This process now turns to the use of another energy source known as *creatine phosphate* (CP); however, in a few seconds the CP supply is exhausted as well.

Another source of quick energy when oxygen is lacking is *glycogen* (stored energy). When the muscle cell is not getting enough oxygen, the breakdown of glycogen extends the ability of a muscle to contract. Once the glycogen breaks down, waste products in the form of *lactic acid* accumulate to the point at which the contraction stops. The final stage of these events is called the *anaerobic phase* or *without oxygen phase* of muscle chemistry, because no oxygen is required. The anaerobic phase can only last a few minutes. For contractions to continue, more oxygen is needed, therefore more supply is required. That supply comes from our nutritional intake. Once the ATP and CP are restored by the nutrients, we enter back into the *aerobic phase* (with oxygen), which releases eighteen times the energy of the anaerobic phase. In most cases of exercise, both phases usually take place simultaneously. Usually one more than the other, but at times both phases are working together, as when you are jogging slow for a long periods.

The human muscle is composed of two types of fiber: *slow-twitch* and *fast-twitch*. The slow-twitch fiber has a higher overall capacity for aerobic energy. Slow-twitch muscle fibers are recruited most during rhythmic endurance exercises, such as running, cycling, or swimming. When you are forced to pedal at full speed, the body then shifts to utilizing fast-twitch fibers. The body now uses less oxygen, allowing for the aerobic/anaerobic phase process explained earlier. Slow-twitch muscle fibers better adapt to physical fitness endurance training, such as walking and cycling.

On the other hand, fast-twitch fibers are specially adapted to short explosive burst of contractions, as when the cyclist mentioned earlier had to pedal full speed. These fast-twitch fibers provide an immediate source of energy when we suddenly run for a bus or up a flight of stairs.

In summary, the interrelationship of the muscular system with the cardiovascular and nervous systems while we exercise is quite exceptional. However, take note: for this vehicle (the human body) to perform properly, we must supply the fuel, and that fuel is balanced nutrition, proper exercise, and sufficient sleep.

Similar to the needs of a performance car engine, gasoline, fluids, oil, water, and rest time are needed. The human body and brain require proteins, fats, carbohydrates, water, movement, and sleep. Would you fuel your sports car by putting sugar in the gas tank or letting it run without oil? Then why would you fill your body with processed sugar or not provide it with the nutrients that are necessary for optimum function? Know what foods you are consuming and their nutritional value. Cheap gas makes for a cheap performance.

# CHAPTER 6

# Assessing your Fitness

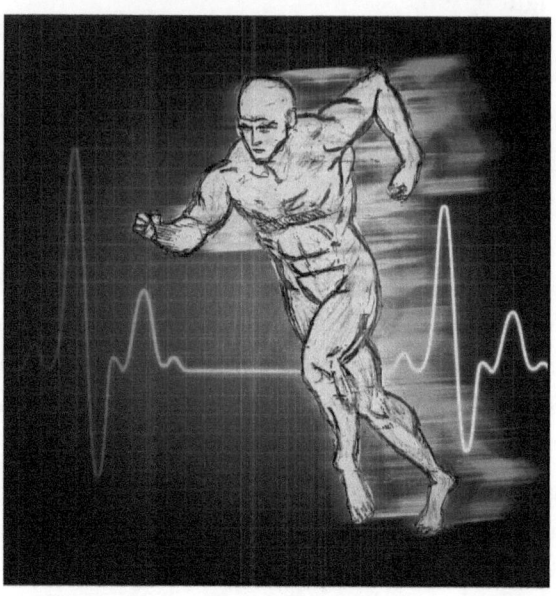

The assessment will provide the basis for setting up an exercise program that is safe, reasonable, and effective. The tests selected measure the health-related components of physical fitness and can be administered with ease and consistency. The tests represent the major areas of fitness evaluation: muscular strength and endurance, cardiorespiratory endurance, and flexibility. Although physical fitness tests have limitations, these recommended tests will provide you with a rough estimate of your physical fitness status. As you complete your assessment, give some thought to the following statements:

- Testing should not dominate your exercise program. Physical fitness measurements will not only help you in evaluating your present condition but will assist you in setting reasonable goals.

- Physical fitness is individual. The intent of self-testing is to help evaluate your present condition and, later on, the effectiveness of your program.
- For those over thirty years old or for anyone who has not recently been active, a medical exam is recommended before attempting these tests or beginning any exercise program.

Physical fitness is more than just bulging muscles or a trim waistline. Although looking good is what most of us want, it does not necessarily reflect our physical fitness. It doesn't matter how good we look or how strong we are, if the heart is unable to meet the circulatory demands of prolonged work, we are not fit. For instance, many men and women appear trim and fit yet tire easily while carrying out their everyday activities.

Each of us is unique, with different abilities in various physical and mental tasks. In addition, we all have our own physiological limitations. Therefore, evaluating physical fitness is a complex matter. However, assessing your fitness level will help you set up a program appropriate for you and your needs. The specific tests selected here for assessing your physical fitness have all been used successfully in recent years to measure the basic levels of physical fitness. They were selected because they provide for uniformity in scoring and overall ease in testing. The tests for the basic physical fitness components have been grouped into the following areas: (a) muscular strength and endurance; (b) flexibility; (c) cardiorespiratory endurance. A reasonable success in all of these tests is necessary for you to be classified as physically fit.

The rationale for the tests and instructions for carrying out each test are presented in the sections that follow.

## Interpreting Your Results

In each section, you will find tables and illustrations that represent test results for young adult men and women who have been involved in physical conditioning programs. These composite scores provide a scale on which you can rate your own performance. These tables do have limitations because of the problems of interpreting and equating the results for all body types and ages. Nevertheless, although these scales cannot give exact values of strengths and weaknesses, they can give you a rough indication of them. If you are low in all tests or only in one or two, consider the reasons why. You may be able to do something about it. Log your results in your twenty-one-day journal for comparison.

## Reasons For Fitness Testing

- Establish one's fitness status
- Use as basis for setting goals
- Use results to design proper workout
- Use to evaluate conditioning changes
- Provide motivation for starting and adhering to an exercise program

## Evaluating Muscular Strength and Endurance

The two fundamental components of physical fitness are muscular strength and muscular endurance. Strength tests have been used as a measure of physical fitness for years because of the relationship between muscular strength and overall physical condition is quite high.

The evaluation procedures here will help you assess your functional strength and endurance. The following strength tests have been used extensively for years and provide reasonable estimates of overall body strength and endurance.

The bent-knee sit-up tests the strength and endurance of the abdominal muscles and, to a limited extent, the hip flexors. Push-ups test the capacities of the arms, chest, and shoulder muscles. Although there are many different test for evaluating fitness these days, the criteria that influence these selections are the ease with which these test can be scored, the simplicity of administering them, and the likelihood of gaining reliable measurements. Remember the purpose of these tests is to get some indication of whether your strength and endurance is low, average, or good.

*Table 7-1* Norms for muscular strength and endurance.

| | Women | Women | Men | Men |
|---|---|---|---|---|
| | Sit-ups (2 minutes) | Push-ups (1 minute) | Sit-ups (2 minutes) | Push-ups (2 minutes) |
| | 66+ | 38+ | 85+ | 54+ |
| **Exceptional** | 62 | 34 | 79 | 50 |
| | 58 | 30 | 73 | 46 |
| | 56 | 28 | 70 | 44 |
| **Excellent** | 54 | 26 | 67 | 42 |
| | 52 | 24 | 63 | 40 |
| | 50 | 22 | 61 | 38 |
| **Good** | 48 | 20 | 59 | 36 |
| | 46 | 18 | 56 | 34 |
| | 44 | 16 | 53 | 32 |
| **Average** | 42 | 14 | 50 | 30 |
| | 40 | 12 | 46 | 28 |
| | 38 | 10 | 44 | 26 |
| **Fair** | 36 | 8 | 41 | 24 |
| | 34 | 6 | 38 | 22 |
| | 32 | 4 | 35 | 20 |
| **Poor** | 30 | 2 | 32 | 18 |
| | 28 | 1 | 29 | 16 |
| | 26 | 0 | 26 | 14 |
| **Very Poor** | 22 | 0 | 20 | 10 |
| | 18 | 0 | 17 | 6 |

*\* For modified push-ups use these scores until you can do full push-ups (See Illustration 7-3)*

# Sit-ups (bent knee)

*Purpose*: To determine the strength and endurance of the abdominal muscles and the hip flexors.

*Procedure*: Assume a supine position (on your back) with hands interlocked behind your neck or with arms folded across the chest. When supporting the back of your neck with your hands, be sure to point elbows forward and lift from your upper body with your abdominal muscles. Do not pull on your neck. Draw your feet back toward the buttocks until they are flat on the floor (knees bent). The angle of your legs to your thighs should be about 90 degrees. It is beneficial to have a partner holding both of your ankles down or lock your feet under a stable surface (bed or sofa). A full sit-up is counted when you have lifted your back and raised your trunk until the lower back is at least perpendicular to the floor and then have returned to the starting position. Repeat this as many times as possible within the time limit. The score is the number of proper sit-ups done in a two-minute time period. Resting is permitted on your back with hands in the proper position.

*Improper procedure:* Not coming all the way up to the vertical position (do not let your elbows touch the knees; your elbows should pass the knees). Also releasing your hands from behind the neck or removing your crossed arms from your chest (do not count these).

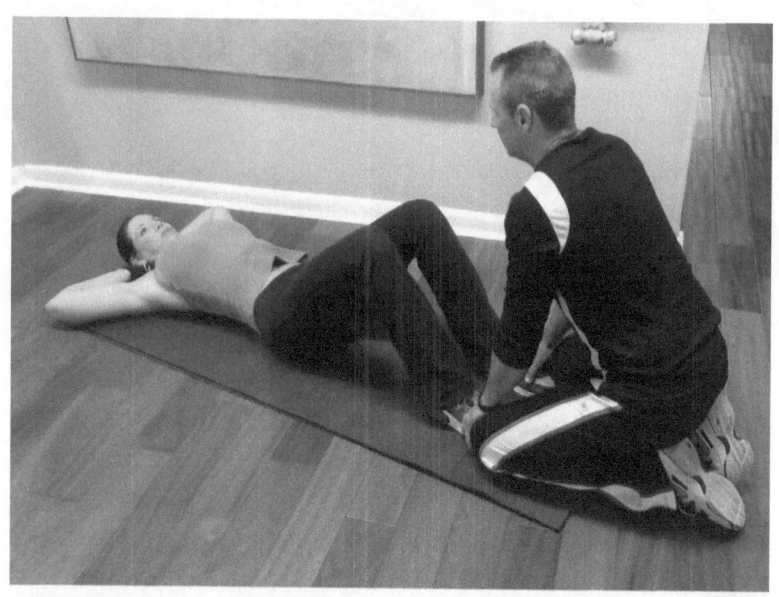

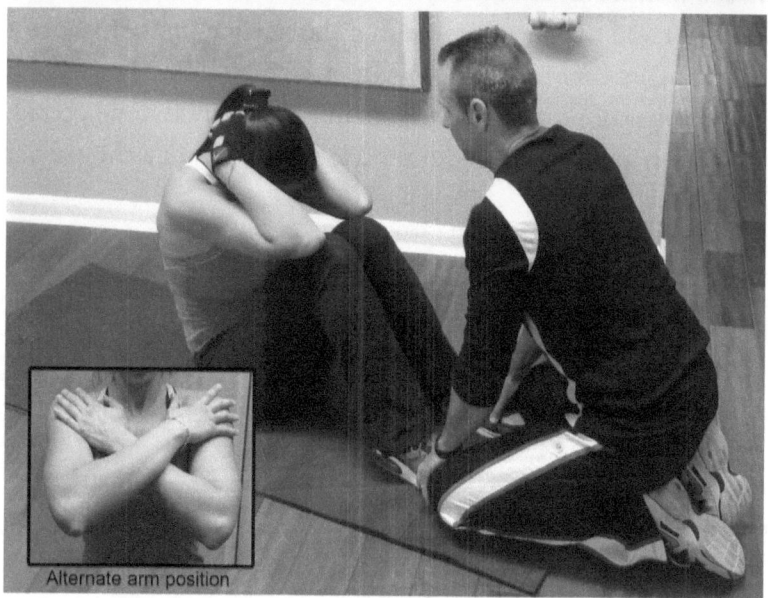

Alternate arm position

*Illustration 7-1*

## Push-up test

*Purpose:* To test the strength and endurance of the flexors of the arms, shoulder girdle, and upper back muscles.

*Procedure*: Kneel on all fours, hands shoulder-width apart, positioned beneath the shoulders. Extend your legs back, weight on the toes, with your body in a straight line (see illustration 7-2). Slowly bend your elbows and lower your torso as a unit until your chest is two inches from the floor. Keeping your back straight, push back up to straight-arm position. Repeat this procedure for one minute.

*Improper procedure*: Not keeping the body straight, allowing it to sag or peak upward. Not going down to two to four inches from the floor or failure to fully straighten arms when pushing back up (do not count these).

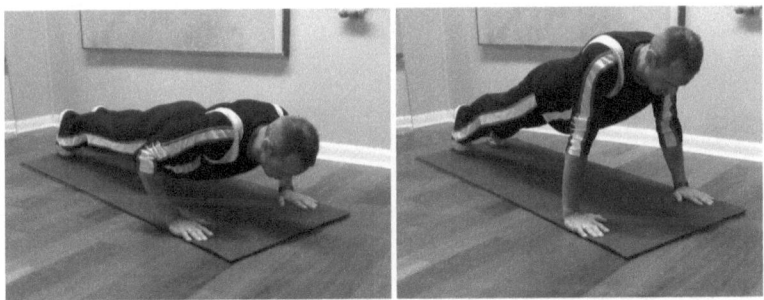

*Illustration 7-2*

*To be used if you are unable to perform one full push-up*

\*Modified push-up

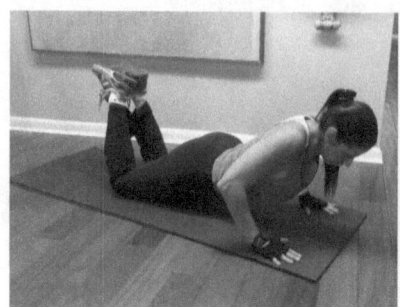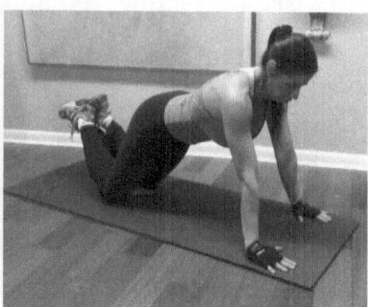

*Illustration 7-3*

*Refer back to table 7-1 for your score and document your results on your profile for later reference.*

## Evaluating Flexibility

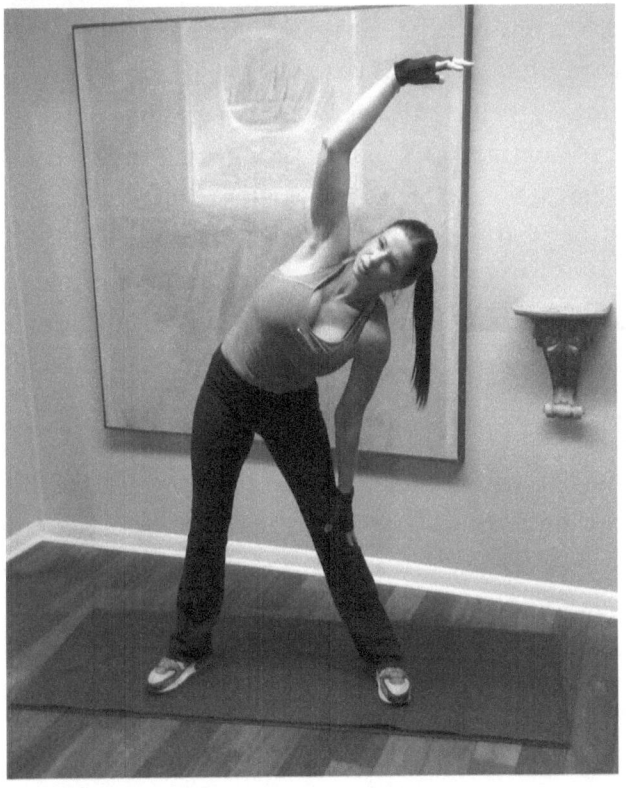

Flexibility is the ability to use a muscle throughout its maximum range of motion. The loss of the ability to bend, twist, and stretch is often a result of muscle disuse, such as in excessive periods of sitting or standing.

Sedentary lifestyles can lead to shortened muscles and tendons, lower back and hip pain, and an imbalance in strength of opposing pairs of muscles. For example, the shortening of the hamstrings is a very common disorder that can be caused by long periods of sitting or standing. This can lead to loss of flexibility in these muscles, which can limit your ability to walk smoothly, to sit or stand up gracefully, and to perform efficiently with everyday tasks. Now let us look at the basic physiology of stretching. Your muscles are protected by a mechanism called the *stretch reflex*. If you stretch the muscle fibers too far (by bouncing or over stretching), a nerve reflex responds by sending a signal to the muscle to contract; this shortens the muscle and keeps it from being injured. Therefore, if you stretch too far, you tighten the muscle that you are trying to stretch. You can avoid this stress reflex issue by *not* overstretching and *not* bouncing into the stretches. Stretching, when done correctly, does not hurt. Learn to pay attention to your body when exercising; pain is an indication that something is wrong.

Stretching exercises should be performed through the full range of motion on a regular basis, using both the *extensors,* the muscles that increase the angle at a joint, and the *flexors,* which decrease the angle. A balanced flexibility program will do the following things:

- Promote circulation
- Increase range of motion
- Reduce muscle and mental tension
- Improve coordination and balance
- Help prevent injuries, such as muscle strains or tendon and ligament tears
- Help relieve muscular pain due to a sedentary lifestyle or overworked lifestyle
- Reduce stress and anxiety

Although no single test will provide adequate information about the flexibility of all major joints of the body, the following two tests provide a reasonable indication of your ability to stretch. *Tables 7-2 and 7-3* provide you with rating for flexibility.

## Trunk Flexion Test

*Purpose:* To measure the amount of trunk flexion and the ability to stretch the back muscles and hamstrings (back thigh muscles).

*Procedure:* It is helpful to have a partner assist with this test. *(Illustration 7-4)* Sit with your legs fully extended and the bottom of your feet flat against a box at least six inches from the wall. Now extend (stretch) your arms and hands forward as far as possible and hold for a count of three while your partner uses a ruler to measure the distance (in inches) between the board and your fingertips. Distances before the edge (not able to reach your toes) are expressed as negative scores and those beyond the edge are expressed as positive scores. See *Table 7-2: Norms for Trunk Flexion (inches from finger tips to bottom of feet).*

*Improper Procedure:* Not holding the flex position for the count of three and bending at the knees.

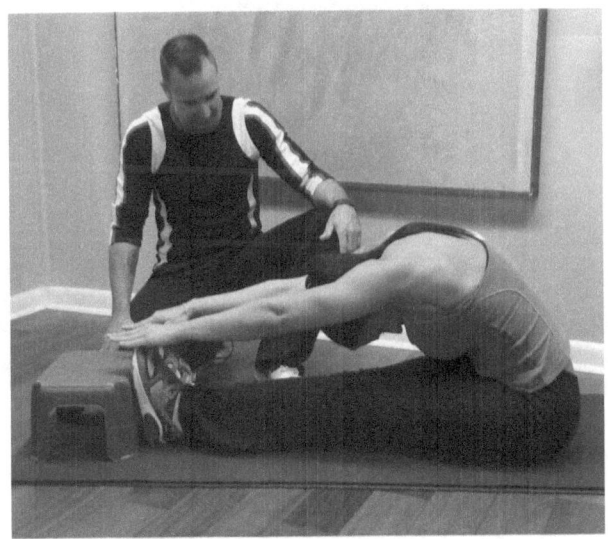

*Illustration 7-4: Trunk Extension*

# Trunk Extension Test

*Purpose:* To measure the range of motion (flexibility) of the back

*Procedure:* Lie in a prone position (face down) on the floor. Have a partner kneel and straddle your legs to hold your buttocks and legs down. With your hands grasped behind your neck, raise your upper trunk (chest and head) off the floor and hold for a count of three. Another person can measure the distance from your chin to the floor. For results see *Table 7-3*.

*Improper Procedure:* Not holding the measuring device in a perpendicular position while measuring. Raising the hips off the floor or not holding the extended position for a count of three.

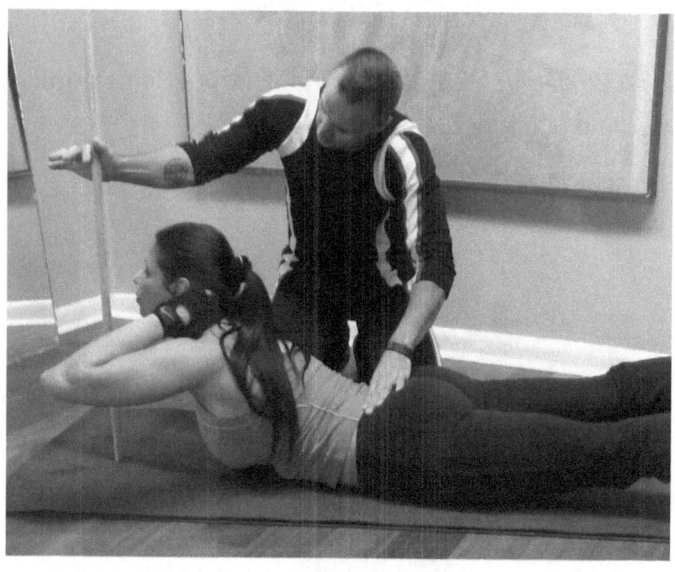

*Illustration 7-5: Trunk Extension*

|              | Women    | Men      |
|--------------|----------|----------|
| Poor range   | 12       | 4        |
| Average      | 21       | 15       |
| Desired range| 21 to 25 | 15 to 20 |

*Table 7-3: Norms for Trunk Extension (inches from chin to floor)*

## Evaluating Cardiorespiratory Endurance

Your cardiovascular health is determined by the ability of the heart to pump blood, of the lungs' capacity to supply oxygen to the rest of the body, and of the muscles to utilize oxygen. All are measures of cardiovascular fitness. Sustained muscular activity is possible only through the effective functioning of the heart, blood vessels, and lungs.

Continuous and rhythmic activities that can be sustained for twenty minutes or more are best for improving the function of the cardiorespiratory system. Walking is the easiest exercise mode to begin with. Running, cycling, swimming, and other continuous exertions can provide added benefits for developing cardiovascular fitness.

Tests involving vigorous physical movement have been devised as sound measures of cardiorespiratory health and endurance. Please consult your health care provider before performing this test. For the purpose of this fitness program, we will use the Step Test heart rate recovery test.

The Step Test is a useful procedure for assessing cardiovascular fitness by measuring the heart rate recovery time. Stepping on and off a bench (sixteen to eighteen inches in height) for a three- to five-minute period at a selected cadence has long been used for rating a person's physical capacity for hard work and evaluating the effects of training. Although the Step Test is not the best predictor of cardiovascular fitness, the heart rate during recovery from a standardized Step Test is an easy way to self-evaluate the heart's response to exercise. *The faster the heart rate recovers after the timed Step Test, the higher your fitness rating.*

This test is easy to perform, takes little time, and does not require special skills. This test does, however, require minimum equipment: a step, locker room bench, bleachers, or just a sturdy wooden box; a watch; and the following chart to record your Step Test results.

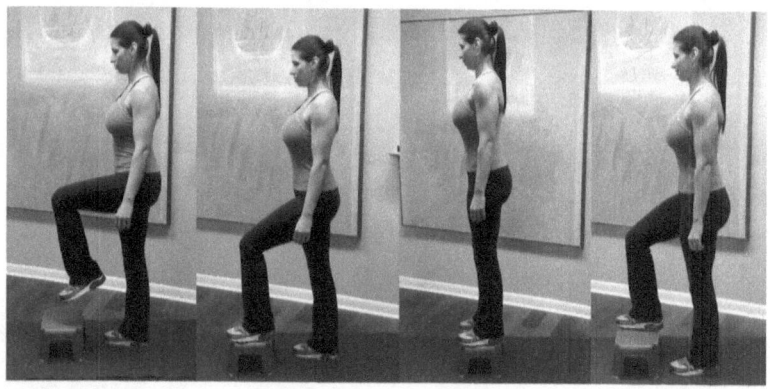

*Illustration 7-6: Step Test*

## Step Test

*Procedure:*

1. A locker room bench (generally sixteen to eighteen inches high) is recommended for both men and women. A bleacher (usually sixteen inches high) can be used, but if neither is available, a sturdy chair or bench at least twelve to eighteen inches high can be used.

2.  You can work with a partner or on your own. Begin when the watch is started, and you start stepping onto the step or chair: first the left foot up, and then the right foot up; then the left foot down and the right foot down. This complete step represents four counts. (You are allowed to change the "up" foot during the test.) Step to the following cadence: one hundred and twenty counts per minute or thirty complete step executions per minute (One four-count step every two seconds: up, up, down, down).

3.  Continue the test for three minutes, keeping the tempo while performing the full step up. (Straighten your knees as you step onto the step, box, or chair.) After stepping for three minutes, stop and sit down.

4.  One minute after the exercise period stops, have your partner or you count your pulse beats for thirty seconds. Log your results. Then record your pulse for the following periods:

    2 to 2.5 minutes after

    3 to 3.5 minutes after

    Count your pulse for each thirty-second period and document the results in the "recording your Step Test results" box (Step Test Log).

*Improper Procedure:*

Not keeping the cadence of thirty step executions per minute
Failure to straighten the knees to full extension on the up steps
Not counting the pulse accurately

*Scoring:* The sum of the three thirty-second pulse measurements is your recovery index. Record your results for each recovery pulse in the Step Test box. Be sure to mark the time of day and the date. Refer to this when you repeat the Step Test at a later date.

The scores will give you some indication of the functional ability of your heart. Use your initial recovery index as your starting point. As you continue your physical conditioning program, you can compare your results to check your progress. This is not a competition. This is basically just keeping score for you.

Be sure to repeat the test under similar conditions: time of day, temperature, no physical activity prior to testing, and so on. As your heart and muscles become better conditioned, your recovery index (the sum of the three recovery measurements) will decrease. This indicates a quicker recovery. Recovery indexes falling below 150 are good scores. Record all of your assessment results in the fitness profile box and refer back to it to compare your progress.

# Recording your step test results

Name: _____ age: _____

STEP TEST

Time: _____ Length: _____ min.

Stepping rate: _____ counts/min.

1 to 1.5 min. _____ Re-eval. _____
2 to 2.5 min. _____        _____
3 to 3.5 min. _____        _____

Total _____ (recovery index)

Date: _____

Time: _____ Bench height: _____ in.

Re-evaluation:

Date: _____

Time: _____ Length _____ min.

Stepping rate: _____ counts/min.

Total _____ (recovery index)

*Step Test Log

FITNESS PROFILE

| Name: | Date: | |
|---|---|---|
| Age: | Height: | Weight: |

| MUSCULAR STRENGTH AND ENDURANCE | | RATING |
|---|---|---|
| Sit-ups: | | |
| Push-ups: | | |

| FLEXIBILITY TEST | | RATING |
|---|---|---|
| Trunk flexion: | inches (+ or -) | |
| Trunk extension: | inches (+ or -) | |

| CARDIORESPIRATORY STEP TEST | | STEPPING RATE |
|---|---|---|
| Total recovery index: | | |

| REEVALUATION | DATE: | |
|---|---|---|
| Sit-ups: | | |
| Push-ups: | | |
| Trunk flexion: | | |
| Trunk extension: | | |

| STEP TEST | | STEPPING RATE |
|---|---|---|
| Total recovery index: | | |

# Conditioning the Physical Body

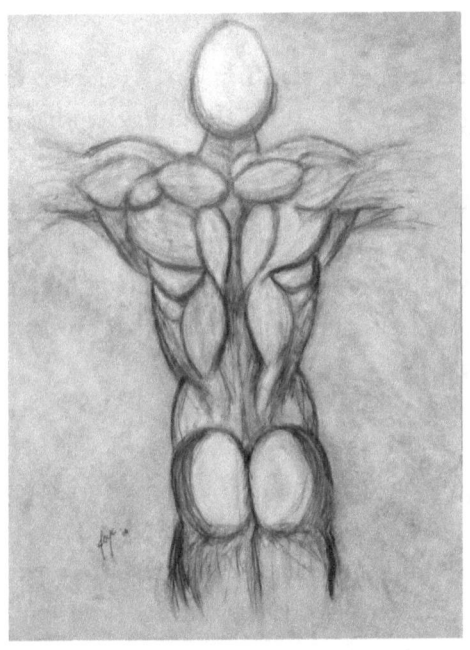

*Lack of activity destroys the good condition
of every human being, while movement and
methodical exercise save it and preserve it.*
*~ Plato*

A balanced physical conditioning program should include: strength and cardiovascular conditioning, a balance and flexibility program, balanced nutrition, and sufficient water and sleep. This may seem like a lot of work, but if you start with the three cornerstones—sufficient sleep, balanced nutrition, and proper movement—the rest will fall into place. The three physical components—strength training, cardiovascular conditioning, and balanced flexibility training—can be mixed and matched. It is best to perform all three components in one session and in a specific order, but they can be done in different sessions and even on different days.

For example, strength training on Monday, cardiovascular conditioning on Tuesday, and flexibility work on Wednesday, take Thursday off, and begin the cycle again on Friday. Or you could do your strength training in the a.m., the cardiovascular conditioning in the p.m., and the flexibility work on the following day. The physical conditioning can be structured or it could be very flexible and spontaneous. Find what works best for your needs and goals.

Now that you have assessed your fitness levels in all areas, it is time to design your personalized exercise program. Your fitness program should be designed based on your current fitness level. Refer back to your test scores in each area. Your exercise program and goals should reflect your current fitness levels. Now you can design the proper program for each component. Keep in mind, your fitness level could vary. For example, you may have scored well on the strength and muscular endurance tests but poorly on the cardiorespiratory evaluation. In this particular scenario, you would begin the strength program at an intermediate level and the cardiovascular conditioning at a beginner level. Progress slowly and mindfully.

Before we get to specific exercises, it is time to set your body improvement goals. We will be using the SMART goal strategy.[24]

---

[24]   Gavin, Lifestyle Fitness Coaching, humankinetics.com.

This will help you set clear and realistic goals. Use the following example to help set your personalized SMART goals:

Example:

- *S = Specifically*: I improve my physical, mental, and spiritual health.
- *M= Measurable:* I drop one pants size and reduce my body fat percentage. I learn something new every day. I try each day to be the best that I can be.
- *A = Action:* I log my progress and begin a gratitude journal. I follow a sensible diet and commit to exercising three times per week. I practice patience and compassion. I begin to learn one new skill. I write a daily to-do list to reduce procrastination and become more productive.
- *R = Reasonable:* I feel and look better. I am slowly improving myself by adding more and more positive habits, (sleeping and resting more, drinking more water, thinking positive, exercising daily, etc.).
- *T = Timely:* I intend to lose at least three pounds in twenty-one days (log date).

*Below is space for you to set your smart goals for twenty-one-day challenge.*

| Name: | Date: |
|---|---|

S = Specifically-

M = Measurable-

A = Action-

R = Realistically-

T = Time frame-

Now that you have set your goals, review them again to make sure they can be accomplished in twenty-one days. Keep in mind, the goals for the twenty-one-day challenge should be realistic for that time frame. Short-term goals are designed to be met within days to weeks. Long-term goals are months to years.

Once you have completed the challenge, you can then set longer-term goals. I recommend setting weekly to monthly goals because this allows you to achieve your desired outcome one step at a time. This allows you to avoid feeling overwhelmed and disappointed. Each time a goal is achieved, it builds confidence and will power, and activates chemicals that give you more motivation to press on. Eventually, short-term goals lead to long-term goals.

At times, life delivers challenges, which include speed bumps that can and will affect your plan of action. Deal with the challenges as best as possible and modify your plan accordingly. Get back to your original plan as soon as possible. If the challenges create long-term changes to your schedule or lifestyle, modify your goals to fit your new schedule. Your goals must work with your lifestyle; otherwise the speed bumps will eventually cause failure in obtaining your goals.

The following list has been broken down into three components: strength, cardiovascular, and flexibility. These are just some examples of exercises that could be integrated into your personalized program. Now that you have assessed your fitness and set up SMART goals appropriate to your current fitness levels, it is time to establish your plan of action. First, set a date to start. Second, choose one exercise from each component listed below or follow one of sample workouts at the end of the chapter. Remember, the workout is designed to improve the entire human system: brain, body, and spirit. Design your plan of action in the space provided at the end of this section and move on to the next chapter.

## Developing Strength and Muscular Endurance

Recommended: 20-40 minutes, 3 to 5 times per week

Strength Programs Could Include:

- Core conditioning
- Free-weight strength training

- Resistance machine training
- Isometric exercises
- Pilates
- Strength yoga
- Swiss ball and resistance band exercises
- Weight bar classes (Power Pump)
- *Rock climbing and mountain biking
- *Kayaking, rowing, white-water rafting, and surfing
  (*These activities have both strength and cardiovascular benefits)

## Developing Balanced Flexibility

Recommended: 10-30 minutes, 3-5 times per week

Flexibility Program Could Include:

- Basic stretching
- Hatha yoga
- Flow yoga
- Pilates
- Tai Chi
- Martial arts

Nonphysical Activities that Help Relax Tense Muscles:

- Massages
- Warm baths/hot tub
- Soothing instrumental music
- Scented candles (chamomile, lavender, or sandalwood)
- Meditation

# Improving Cardiorespiratory Endurance

Recommended: When performed in fusion format, 5-10 minutes per day, 3-5 days per week. When cardio is done on its own, 30-45 minutes is recommended.

Cardiovascular Programs Could Include:

- Walking, jogging, or running
- Cycling or swimming
- Aerobic classes
- Other cardiovascular equipment, such as the elliptical trainer or stair climber (just to name a few)
- Tennis
- Racquetball
- Sports such as football, baseball, soccer, and basketball
- Diving and gymnastics
- Boxing, karate, and other martial arts
- Flow yoga
- Walking your dog, cleaning the house, or cutting your grass (all movement counts with the proper duration of twenty-plus minutes)

All three components of the physical conditioning are recommended. The Joyefit Fusion was designed with brain chemistry in mind. The program is structured to first activate some warming chemicals, such as norepinephrine (noradrenaline), endorphins, and dopamine, which increase motivation, energy, and, to some degree, pleasure. As norepinephrine (noradrenalin) increases the stress hormones, adrenaline and cortisol begin to decrease. The second portion of the workout is focused strength training. This further reduces the stress hormones (adrenaline and cortisol) while activating cooling chemicals, such as acetylcholine and serotonin. The third portions is followed by flexibility, focus, and balance work to activate more of the cooling chemicals, such as GABA and endorphins, improving mood and reducing physical and mental tension. The final portion of the workout is quiet time (meditation). At this point, the workout is activating the release of more cooling chemicals, such as endorphins, GABA, and oxytocin, or vasopressin in men. Follow the protocol in this order: warm up, strength training, and cardiovascular conditioning; then end with flexibility, balance work, and quiet time. In addition, after the quiet time, you can count your blessings by writing three to five things that you are grateful for and why. This work at the end of the workout continues to activate more cooling chemicals, improving your mood, relieving stress, and reducing mental and physical tension. The fusion protocol utilizes exercises that stimulate rewarding warming (SNS) chemicals in the beginning of the workout (raising the heart rate), and ending the workout with exercises that stimulate cooling (PNS) stress reducing chemicals, (lowering the heart rate). The following sample workouts have been provided to begin the twenty-one-day challenge. Choose one that fits your needs and goals or design your own program in the space provided in the next section (Plan of Action Log). Otherwise, implement one of the sample programs listed below.

## The Joyefit *Fusion* Workout

Exercise Structured to Improve the Entire Human System

**Beginner Program** (30 minutes, 3 times per week)

- 15 minutes walking, jogging, cycling, or swimming
- 10 minutes core conditioning, flexibility, and balance work (Pilates, stretch, and yoga balance poses)

- 5 minutes mindfulness/quiet time
- Gratitude (write 3 per day)
- Goals/intentions (write 3 per day)

## Intermediate Program (60 minutes, 4 times per week)

- 5 minutes walking (warm up)
- 15 minutes strength training, total body: lower body on one day and upper body on the next (free weights, resistance bands, or machines)
- 20 minutes cardiovascular conditioning (cycling, walking, running, swimming, or any continuous rhythmic activity)
- 5 minutes core conditioning exercises (Pilates or Swiss ball core exercises)
- 10 minutes yoga and balance work
- 5 minutes mindfulness/quiet time
- Gratitude (write 5 per day and why)
- Goals/intentions (write 5 per day)

The Joyefit Fusion workout is designed to be performed in this specific order. However, if your time is limited, the program can be broken up into several sessions.

For example: This split routine can be done separately 3 times per week.

## Morning Workout #1 (30 minutes)

- 5 minutes warm up
- 15 minutes strength training
- 10 minutes cardiovascular conditioning
- Gratitude list, times 5

**Evening Workout #2** (35 minutes)

- 20 minutes cardiovascular conditioning
- 10 minutes yoga and balance work
- 5 minutes core conditioning

The workouts can also be performed on alternating days. For example: workout #1 on Monday, workout #2 on Tuesday, skip Wednesday, and repeat #1 on Thursday and #2 on Friday.

For additional motivation, inspiration, and support, visit www.joyefit.com for the *advanced,* trademarked Joyefit Fusion workout DVD package. Johnny O will guide you through the fusion workout with clear instructions, continuous flow, motivation, and inspiration.

*Example:*

| Plan Of Action | |
|---|---|
| | Start Date: |
| **DESIGN AND STRUCTURE THE THREE PHYSICAL COMPONENTS** | |
| *Total Body with free weights* | -Strength training |
| *Walking or cycling* | -Cardiovascular conditioning |
| *Yoga* | -Balance and flexibility training |
| *Meditation & Gratitude journal* | -Mindful and spiritual discipline |
| | |
| Additional: *Workout for one hour 3 times per week and stay active on the other days of the week. Follow a sensible balanced diet. Meditate for 5-10 minutes 3 times per week and write 3 things that I'm grateful for and why 5 times per week.* | |
| | |
| | |

Once you complete Part III, apply your plan of action into the twenty-one-day journal (located at the end of Part III), and begin the challenge.

Now that you have set your plan of action for the physical component, we can now move on to the nutritional review. This chapter will explain the importance of each nutrient and help you design a meal plan specifically for your goals.

# CHAPTER 8

# Nutrition

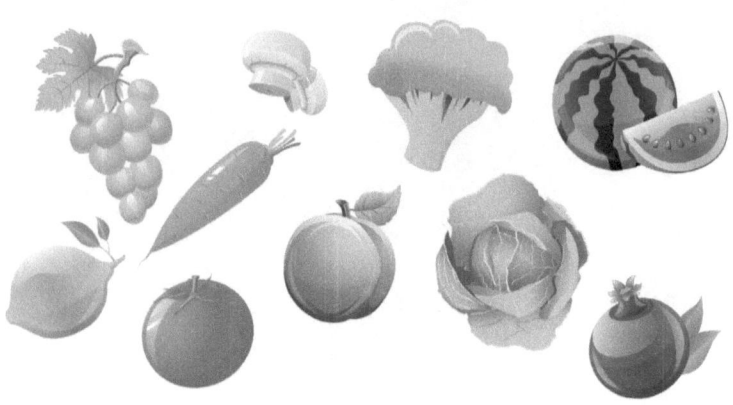

*Let food be thy medicine and medicine be thy food.*
*~ Hippocrates*

Remember the three cornerstones to optimum brain and body function are balanced nutrition, proper exercise, and sufficient sleep. This chapter will cover the information that will help you create a balanced nutrition program for you and your family. Now let's explore the raw details of nutrients.

Nutrients are the raw materials needed for optimum health. Those raw materials are derived from the nutrition that we consume. The nutrients that we receive come from the foods that we eat and the fluids that we drink. Nutrients fall into six categories, all found in most foods.

The nutrient water is the most predominant. The three energy nutrients—carbohydrates, fats, and protein—are next in abundance. Last are the vitamins and minerals, in smaller yet significant amounts.

These nutrients are the construction materials for the maintenance, regulation, and rebuilding of the human cells, muscles, and tissues. That includes all of the functions and processes of the brain.

### The Six Nutrient Categories and Their Physiological Functions Within the Body

| *NUTRIENT* | *FUNCTIONS* |
|---|---|
| *Proteins* | *Builds & repairs mind & body Tissue* |
| *Carbohydrates* | *Provides energy for the brain and the body* |
| *Fats* | *Necessary part of every cell, protects internal organs and carries fat soluble vitamins* |
| *Water* | *Regulates mind & body processes Important for the many chemical reactions of the brain and the body* |
| | |

Before we get into the specifics of each nutrient, I would like to give you a few helpful tips:

- The marketing of food is designed to make you think that you need that product; they even go to the extreme of placing processed foods at eye level, with fancy packaging. Be cautious about all processed foods (most foods that come in a box or bag are more than likely processed with additives).

- Check the nutritional value on all foods: look at the nutritional labels and check the servings per package (the nutritional numbers on the labels are per serving). One package could have five servings, which means five times the number on the label.
- Never shop hungry and always write a list. Stick to the list!
- Shop the perimeter of the stores first; this is where all the fresh fruits, vegetables, meats, fish, and dairy will be. Stock up on the whole foods first and then proceed to the aisles with all the processed foods.
- Avoid the aisle with candy, cookies, and crackers. This can be a weakness for most, including myself. I avoid that aisle like a plague.
- Be careful at the checkout. This is where they set another trap. The sweets are now at your fingertips, but you can work on your will power by not blowing it at the last minute. If need be, grab a pack of sugar-free gum or read a tabloid until you are away from the threat.
- Each time that you leave the store without caving in to your sugar craving, give yourself credit. Go home and write down "I did it. I am in control of my eating, and sugar does not control me." Your brain will remember this reinforcement and it will become easier each time.

*Now for more specifics of each nutrient and why we need them:*

## a) Protein

Protein is considered to be the building block of all bodily components, including muscle, hair, enzymes, and hormones. These proteins are made up of amino acids. These amino acids fuel, repair, and rebuild the brain and the body. The quality of protein is determined by its balance of amino acids. Protein that is higher in quality is more efficiently utilized and better absorbed, which makes us need less. The human body requires twenty different amino acids for optimum performance; nine of them are *essential:* lysine, tryptophane, methionine, valine, leucine, isoleucine, histidine, threonine, and phenylalanine. Since our bodies cannot make these, they must be ingested from our diets. We are able to produce the remaining amino acids, but it does deplete precious materials and energy during the process, so it is best to consume proteins that are rich in all amino acids.

For this reason, it is important to integrate the input of these proteins into our diets. Animal meats are the most abundant in amino acids. Amino acids create proteins, including tyrosine. Tyrosine is what dopamine and norepinephrine are made from. Choline is a precursor to acetylcholine, and L-glutamine is a precursor of glutamate. All of these proteins repair and rebuild the brain and the body. By increasing our protein intake, we will provide our system with the fuel that it needs to produce more of the neurotransmitters that keep us balanced.

It is, however, important to be selective of the source of protein that we eat. Many protein sources are also high in saturated fat. These fats are not recommended due to the negative health effects, such as blood and circulatory problems, heart problems, and obesity.

Fish, egg whites, and lean animal meats, such as poultry, turkey, and lean beef are recommended. If you are someone who likes to try new things, other meats such as quail, pheasant, buffalo, elk, antelope, and venison are all a good source of protein. I also recommend protein powders and shakes made of whey protein, egg protein, or soy protein. Whey protein is dairy-based and is my preferred choice because it is absorbed rapidly. Egg protein is another excellent source and is good for those that are lactose intolerant. Soy protein is a vegetable protein, but since it is fibrous and long-lasting (not absorbed as quickly), it is better used as a meal replacement. When possible try to eat meats that are free-range, with no additives or hormones. Now the question may be, how much protein do we require per day? That is a question that has been debated in the science community for over one hundred years. There are several reasons why it has been difficult to reach a consensus on protein intake. The first is that the amount of protein required by each individual is based on several things, such as age, weight, and activity level. I would include stress level as well, although I don't have the scientific evidence to prove it, but I do believe that stress depletes us of nutrients and proteins. Your protein intake depends on your specific activity level, the intensity of the activity, your body weight, and your age. For example, an endurance athlete or one in strength sports could use more protein because protein can act like a reserve fuel tank supplying amino acids to fuel the brain and body when it is depleted. Consider protein the construction material that strengthens the brain and the body; you cannot build without it. The approximate daily protein requirement for your needs can be figured using this basic formula provided by the American Council on Exercise. Use the number of your current weight, divided by 2.2 (kg), multiplied by 1.5 (lbs.).[25] For example, if you were to weigh 150 pounds divided by 2.2, equals 68.18, times 1.5, equals 103. Therefore, the daily protein recommendation for this scenario is approximately 103 grams of protein per day. Protein provides the building blocks for human cells and includes repairing and rebuilding the health of the brain. Carbohydrates and fats are equally important in keeping optimum health and performance, but in my opinion, protein is

---

[25]    ACE PT Certification, American Council on Exercise, www.acefitness.org.

the most important nutrient for the balance and regulation of the brain and the physical body. A protein source should be included in every meal and supplemented if needed to meet your specific protein requirement. We must also consider that nutritional intake is determined by caloric expenditure. Therefore, the intake of all nutrients should be increased as expenditure increases. For instance, if your activity level increases, so should your nutritional intake of protein, carbohydrates, and fats. Consider protein to be the construction crew that lays the foundation for the roads to your super highway to strength and balance. Now we can move on to the basics and importance of carbohydrates.

## b) Carbohydrates

During digestion, carbohydrates are broken down into glucose. Glucose circulates in the blood, where it is known as blood sugar. The blood sugar is now used by the brain, the body, and the nervous system as energy. If brain cells are deprived of glucose, mental and physical function will suffer. Glucose is also converted into glycogen for storage in either the muscles or the liver. About two-thirds of the body's glycogen is stored in the muscles, and one-third in the liver. As muscles use glycogen, it is broken back down into glucose. Carbohydrates are in just about everything that we eat. Although carbohydrates do not contain any fat, if you consume more than you need or can utilize, they will ultimately be stored as body fat. Among the nutrients, carbohydrates are the most powerful in affecting energy levels and are the body's favorite source of energy. In fact, the body prefers to burn carbohydrates over protein and fat. The best sources of carbohydrates are natural foods, such as fruits, vegetables, and whole grains. These natural foods are rich in antioxidants and other vitamins and minerals. Most are absorbed slowly and do not cause blood sugar spikes.

(See *Chart 1-1: The Glycemic Index* for a detailed rating of foods and the relative ability to spike blood sugar levels.) Minimize the carbohydrates that cause blood sugar spikes. Avoid the foods that are high on the glycemic index. This index was created to help us make better choices so we don't spike our blood sugar to dangerous levels that could lead to diabetes, circulatory problems, or heart complications. Use the index to keep you in line. About 40 percent of your daily caloric consumption should consist of carbohydrates, such as whole grains, beans, fruits, and vegetables. Avoid processed carbohydrates that increase spikes in blood sugar and additional storage of body fat. Limit or avoid processed foods and simple sugars, such as table sugar, sodas, sugar drinks, cakes, cookies, candy, crackers, chips, alcohol, and complex carbohydrates in the form of white potatoes, white pasta, white bread, and white rice. When possible, stick to whole grain breads and pastas, brown rice, and sweet potatoes for a good source of complex carbohydrates. For body improvement purposes, avoid high-glycemic carbohydrates in your last meal of the day, and replace them with two low-glycemic vegetables or fruits. Keep in mind that a serving is about the size of your palm, and approximately five servings per day should provide you with the needed fuel for optimum health and performance. Fuel the mind and body when needed, and modify as your activity level changes.

The more calories that you burn, the more will be needed to provide that energy. The glycemic index is provided to help you determine which carbohydrates are best for your specific meal plan. Choose your carbs wisely and for the purpose of nutritional needs and not emotional needs. Also keep in mind the nutritional ratio of carbohydrates at about 40 percent of your total calories. For example, a daily intake of two thousand calories would allow for eight hundred of those calories to be derived from carbohydrates. And of those eight hundred calories, the total grams of carbohydrates should not exceed three hundred grams per day. Fuel the mind and body when needed and when the most energy is required. Think of it this way: you are fasting during sleep with no nutrients or water for many hours, so the first thing you should do in the morning is provide the body with a healthy balance of protein, fats, and carbohydrates. This means that in order to feel and do your best, breakfast is a must. And by eating first thing in the morning, you are revving up your metabolism, which will eventually assist you in burning calories more efficiently throughout the day. Now we can move on to fats.

## c) Fats

A large percentage of brain receptors are made from fats, and the amount of fat in your diet has a direct impact on the responsiveness of those receptors. But be aware that not all fats are created equal. Fatty acids are the molecular components of fats and oils. They come in several categories: saturated, monounsaturated, and polyunsaturated. The main sources of cholesterol-raising fats are saturated fats. For example, dairy, fatty meats, organ meats, some shellfish, and egg yolks are high in cholesterol and should be limited. Saturated fats are also in fried foods, baked foods, and spreads; these foods should also be limited. Replacing these fats with polyunsaturated and monounsaturated fats, such as olive oil, canola oil, seeds, nuts, olives, natural peanut butter, and most fish can help reduce the bad cholesterol and improve the good cholesterol, improving the overall cholesterol profile. Fat is not your enemy; just choose the good fats.

# Glycemic Index

Chart 1-1
Index of Glycemic (Blood-Sugar-Increasing)
Ratings of Selected Food

The following numbers indicate the relative ability of selected foods to raise blood sugar levels. Foods with higher numbers (with glucose being arbitrarily set at the highest, 100) raise blood sugar the quickest.[26]

---

[26]   Garrison and Somer, The Nutrition Desk Reference, Glycemic index.

# Glycemic Index List

| Food: | G.I. | Food: | G.I. |
|---|---|---|---|
| **BAKERY PRODUCTS** | | **LEGUMES** | |
| Cake, sponge | 66 | Soya beans, canned | 20 |
| Cake, banana, made with sugar | 67 | Soya beans | 25 |
| Cake, pound | 77 | Lentils, red | 36 |
| Cake, banana, made without sugar | 79 | Beans, dried, not specified | 40 |
| Pastry | 84 | Lentils, not specified | 41 |
| Pizza, cheese | 86 | Kidney beans | 42 |
| Muffins | 88 | Lentils, green | 42 |
| Cake, flan | 93 | Butter beans + 5 g. sucrose | 43 |
| Cake, angel food | 95 | Butter beans + 10 g. sucrose | 44 |
| Croissant | 96 | Butter beans | 44 |
| Crumpet | 98 | Split peas, yellow, boiled | 45 |
| Donut | 108 | Lima beans, baby, frozen | 46 |
| Waffles | 109 | Chick peas (garbanzo beans) | 47 |
| | | Kidney beans, autoclaved | 49 |
| **BEVERAGES** | | Haricot/navy beans | 54 |
| Soy milk | 43 | Pinto beans | 55 |
| Cordial, orange | 94 | Chick peas, curry, canned | 58 |
| Soft drink, Fanta | 97 | Black-eyed beans | 59 |
| Lucozade | 136 | Chick peas, canned | 60 |
| | | Pinto beans, canned | 64 |
| **BREADS** | | Romano beans | 65 |
| Bürgen Soy Lin | 27 | Baked beans, canned | 69 |
| Bürgen Oat Bran & Honey Loaf | 43 | Kidney beans, canned | 74 |
| Bürgen Mixed Grain | 48 | Lentils, green, canned | 74 |
| Barley kernel bread | 55 | Butter beans + 15 g. sucrose | 77 |
| Bürgen Fruit Loaf | 62 | Beans, dried, P. vulgaris | 100 |
| Holsom's | 64 | Broad beans (fava beans) | 113 |
| Rye Kernel bread | 66 | | |
| Fruit loaf | 67 | **PASTA** | |
| Oat bran bread | 68 | Spaghetti, protein enriched | 38 |
| Mixed grain bread | 69 | Fettuccine | 46 |
| Pumpernickel | 71 | Vermicelli | 50 |
| Bulger bread | 76 | Spaghetti, wholemeal | 53 |
| Linseed rye bread | 78 | Star pastina | 54 |
| Pita bread, white | 82 | Ravioli, durum, meat filled | 56 |
| Hamburger bun | 87 | Spaghetti, boiled 5 min | 52 |
| Rye flour bread | 92 | Spaghetti, white | 59 |
| Semolina bread | 92 | Spiral, durum | 61 |
| Oat kernel bread | 93 | Capellini | 64 |
| Barley flour bread | 95 | Macaroni | 64 |
| Wheat bread, high fiber | 97 | Linguine | 65 |
| Wheat bread, wholemeal flour | 99 | Instant noodles | 67 |
| Melba toast | 100 | Tortellini, cheese | 71 |
| Wheat bread, white | 101 | Spaghetti, durum | 78 |
| Bagel, white | 103 | Macaroni and Cheese | 92 |
| Kaiser rolls | 104 | Gnocchi | 95 |
| Whole-wheat snack bread | 105 | Rice pasta, brown | 131 |
| Bread stuffing | 106 | | |
| Wheat bread, Wonderwhite | 112 | **ROOT VEGETABLES** | |
| Wheat bread, gluten free | 129 | Yam | 73 |
| French baguette | 136 | Sweet potato | 77 |
| | | Potato, white, not specified, boiled | 80 |
| **BREAKFAST CEREALS** | | Potato, new | 81 |
| Rice Bran | 27 | Potato, white, Ontario | 85 |
| Kelloggs' All Bran Fruit 'n Oats | 55 | Potato, canned | 87 |
| Kelloggs' Guardian | 59 | Potato, Prince Edward Island, boiled | 90 |
| All-bran | 60 | Beets | 91 |
| Red River Cereal | 70 | Potato, steamed | 93 |
| Bran Buds | 75 | Potato mashed | 100 |
| Special K | 77 | Carrots | 70 |
| Oat Bran | 78 | Swede (rutabaga) | 103 |
| Kelloggs' Honey Smacks | 78 | Potato, boiled, mashed | 104 |
| Muesli | 80 | French fries | 107 |
| Kelloggs' Mini-Wheats (whole wheat) | 81 | Potato, microwaved | 117 |

| | |
|---|---|
| Bran Chex | 83 |
| Kelloggs' Just Right | 84 |
| Porridge (oatmeal) | 87 |
| Life | 94 |
| Nutri-grain | 94 |
| Grapenuts | 96 |
| Sustain | 97 |
| Shredded Wheat | 99 |
| Kelloggs' Mini-Wheats (blackcurrant) | 99 |
| Cream of Wheat | 100 |
| Wheat Biscuit | 100 |
| Golden Grahams | 102 |
| Pro Stars | 102 |
| Sultana Bran | 102 |
| Puffed Wheat | 105 |
| Cheerios | 106 |
| Corn Bran | 107 |
| Breakfast bar | 109 |
| Total | 109 |
| Cocopops | 110 |
| Post Flakes | 114 |
| Rice Krispies | 117 |
| Team | 117 |
| Corn Chex | 118 |
| Cornflakes | 119 |
| Crispix | 124 |
| Rice Chex | 127 |
| Rice Bubbles | 128 |

## CEREAL GRAINS

| | |
|---|---|
| Barley, pearled | 36 |
| Rye | 48 |
| Wheat kernels | 59 |
| Rice, instant, boiled 1 min | 65 |
| Bulgur | 68 |
| Rice, parboiled | 68 |
| Rice, parboiled, high amylose | 69 |
| Barley, cracked | 72 |
| Wheat, quick cooking | 77 |
| Buckwheat | 78 |
| Sweet corn | 78 |
| Rice, specialty | 78 |
| Rice, brown | 79 |
| Rice, wild, Saskatchewan | 81 |
| Rice, white | 83 |
| Rice, white, high amylose | 83 |
| Couscous | 93 |
| Barley, rolled | 94 |
| Rice, Mahatma Premium | 94 |
| Taco shells | 97 |
| Cornmeal | 98 |
| Millet | 101 |
| Rice, Pelde | 109 |
| Rice, Sunbrown Quick | 114 |
| Tapioca, boiled with milk | 115 |
| Rice, Calrose | 124 |
| Rice, parboiled, low amylose Pelde | 124 |
| Rice, white, low amylose | 126 |
| Rice, instant, boiled 6 min | 128 |

| *COOKIES* | |
|---|---|
| Oatmeal cookies | 79 |
| Rich Tea cookies | 79 |
| Digestives | 84 |
| Shredded Wheatmeal | 89 |
| Shortbread | 91 |
| Arrowroot | 95 |
| Graham Wafers | 106 |
| Vanilla Wafers | 110 |
| Morning Coffee cookies | 113 |

| *CRACKERS* | |
|---|---|

| | |
|---|---|
| Potato, instant | 118 |
| Potato, baked | 121 |
| Parsnips | 139 |

## SNACK FOOD AND CONFECTIONARY

| | |
|---|---|
| Peanuts | 21 |
| Mars M&Ms (peanut) | 46 |
| Mars Snickers Bar | 57 |
| Mars Twix Cookie Bars (caramel) | 62 |
| Mars Chocolate (Dove) | 63 |
| Jams and marmalades | 70 |
| Chocolate | 70 |
| Potato crisps | 77 |
| Popcorn | 79 |
| Muesli Bars | 87 |
| Mars Kudos Whole Grain Bars (choc chip) | 87 |
| Mars Bar | 91 |
| Mars Skittles | 98 |
| Life Savers | 100 |
| Corn chips | 105 |
| Jelly beans | 114 |
| Pretzels | 116 |
| Dates | 141 |

## SOUPS

| | |
|---|---|
| Tomato Soup | 54 |
| Lentil soup, canned | 63 |
| Split pea soup | 86 |
| Black bean soup | 92 |
| Green pea soup, canned | 94 |

## SUGARS

| | |
|---|---|
| Organic Agave Nectar | 14 |
| Fructose | 32 |
| Lactose | 65 |
| Honey | 83 |
| High fructose corn syrup | 89 |
| Sucrose | 92 |
| Glucose | 137 |
| Glucose tablets | 146 |
| Maltodextrin | 150 |
| Maltose | 150 |

## VEGETABLES

| | |
|---|---|
| Peas, dried | 32 |
| Marrowfat, dried | 66 |
| Peas, green | 68 |
| Sweet corn | 78 |
| Pumpkin | 107 |

## FRUIT AND FRUIT PRODUCTS

| | |
|---|---|
| Cherries | 32 |
| Grapefruit | 36 |
| Apricots, dried | 44 |
| Pear, fresh | 53 |
| Apple | 54 |
| Plum | 55 |
| Apple juice | 58 |
| Peach, fresh | 60 |
| Orange | 63 |
| Pear, canned | 63 |
| Grapes | 66 |
| Pineapple juice | 66 |
| Peach, canned | 67 |
| Grapefruit juice | 69 |
| Orange juice | 74 |
| Kiwifruit | 75 |
| Banana | 77 |
| Fruit cocktail | 79 |
| Mango | 80 |
| Sultanas | 80 |
| Apricots, fresh | 82 |

| | | | | |
|---|---|---|---|---|
| Jatz | 79 | Pawpaw | 83 |
| High Fibre Rye Crispread | 93 | Apricots, canned, syrup | 91 |
| Breton Wheat Crackers | 96 | Raisins | 91 |
| Stoned Wheat Thins | 96 | Rockmelon (muskmelon) | 93 |
| Sao | 100 | Pineapple | 94 |
| Water Crackers | 102 | Watermelon | 103 |
| Rice Cakes | 110 | | |
| Puffed Crispbread | 116 | | |
| **DAIRY FOODS** | | | |
| Yogurt, low fat, artificially sweet | 20 | | |
| Milk, chocolate, artifically sweet | 34 | | |
| Milk + 30 g bran | 38 | | |
| Milk, full fat | 39 | | |
| Milk, skim | 46 | | |
| Yogurt, low fat, fruit sugar sweet | 47 | | |
| Milk, chocolate, sugar sweetened | 49 | | |
| Yogurt, unspecified | 51 | | |
| Milk + custard + starch + sugar | 61 | | |
| Yakult (fermented milk) | 64 | | |
| Ice cream, low fat | 71 | | |
| Ice cream | 87 | | |

Please keep in mind that all of the foods listed in the index have some nutritional value. However, the foods with the highest glycemic rating have the fastest spike in blood sugar levels. Those with a lower glycemic rating provide the brain with glucose at a steadier rate and are preferable to foods with a higher glycemic rating.

Simple carbohydrates, such as refined sugars and flour, flood your brain and body with glucose, followed by a crash. Even though the brain gets flooded by glucose for a short period, it is just as suddenly deprived of it and quickly craves more. This is what some call the sugar hangover. In general, most complex carbohydrates, such as sweet potatoes, brown rice, and whole grains, are preferable because of their time-release properties. This gives us steadier and longer-term glucose and therefore more mental and physical energy.

Just as with protein, the timing and portion of your carbohydrates is critical to how your brain will respond. Fuel the brain and the body when it is needed. Timing is everything. The food we consume is the fuel that runs the brain and the body. The proper amount allows for optimum mental/physical function and performance. Use the index as a guide to help you make better choices for the appropriate times. In conclusion, below are some helpful tips to help avoid food traps that are designed to make us eat more than we should.

## Some Helpful Tips

- Out of sight, out of mind. Keep temptation out of your sight, and if need be, do not have those foods in your environment (work, home, etc.).

- If you are having problems achieving your weight loss goals, begin to write a food journal. The twenty-one-day journal provides space for logging your daily food intake. Writing a food log helps you recognize where you can make improvements.

- Beware of external cues, such as marketing in commercials and grocery stores. Candy and cookie aisles in the grocery store are full of external cues that trigger sugar cravings. Food corporations understand what triggers the brain to want something. Be aware of fancy wrapping and boxes, bright colors, foods advertised as light, no sugar added, and sugar-free. Light could mean lighter in color, and no sugar added could still contain high sugar content. Instead, pay attention to your internal cues, such as hunger.

For example: the service staff in most restaurants will remove plates from the table that are either empty or even full of chicken wing bones left from the pile of all-you-can-eat wing night. The plate full of bones is the brain's external cue that you have had enough. If we see the pile of bones, the brain will begin to determine how much has already been eaten, therefore cuing you to back off and eat less.

# Water/ H2O

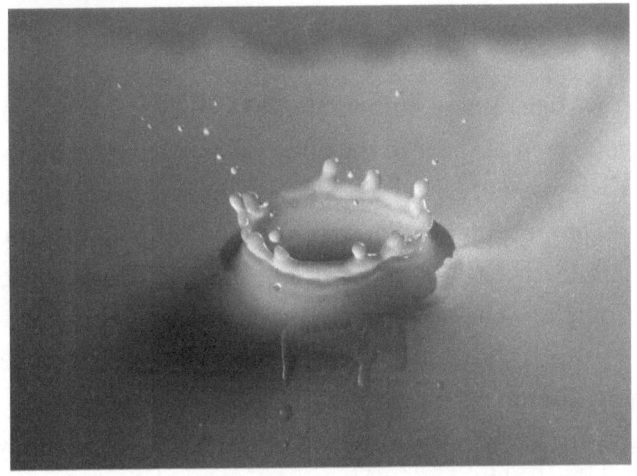

*If there is magic on this planet, it is contained
in water. Without water there is no life.*
*~Loren Eiscley, anthropologist, 1907*

Functions of Water Include:

1.  Body temperature is regulated through the evaporation of water from the skin.
2.  The foods we eat are digested in an abundance of digestive juices (water).
3.  The nutrients are carried in solution across the intestinal walls.
4.  Materials dissolved in water are transported across the cell membranes.
5.  Chemical reactions take place in the presence of water.
6.  Water has a lubricating effect to help avoid friction between body parts.

With the exception of oxygen, water is the most important to life. We can survive for a few weeks without food, but we can only survive a few days without water.

About 50-70 percent of our total body weight is made up of water. The proportion of water in the body varies. Men have more body water than women. Lean bodies have more water than those with a greater proportion of adipose tissue (body fat), and infants and young children have more than older people. Every cell of the body contains water. Blood plasma is about 90 percent water; muscle tissue is about 70-80 percent water; fat tissue is 20 percent and bone about 20 percent. Intracellular fluid (within the cells) accounts for about three-quarters of the water in the body and extracellular fluid (outside the cell).

Water is lost from the body through the kidneys, skin, lungs, and bowels. Usually, most water is lost through urination. Another way that we lose water is through the skin by insensible perspiration. With vigorous activity, especially in warm weather, we lose a larger amount of water through visible perspiration. So basically, the proper intake of water determines the function of the brain and the body. And remember, once you sense thirst, you are already dehydrated. Drink water periodically throughout the day and make it a habit. (The daily recommended amount of water is approximately sixty-four ounces.)

# CHAPTER 9

# Natural Supplements

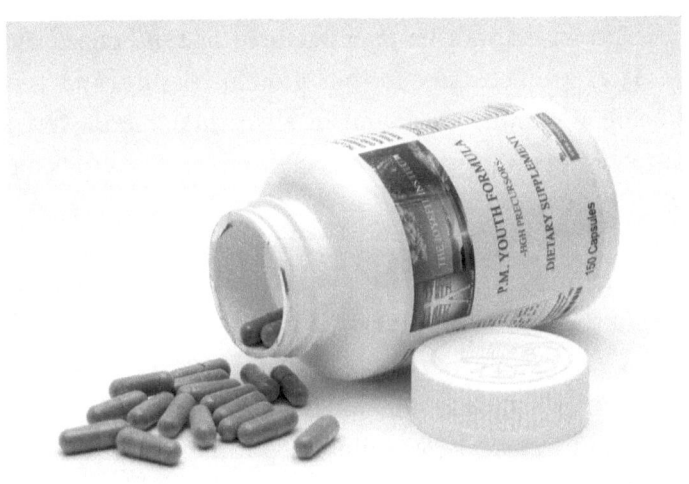

*The Earth's natural substances are the true healers of disease.*
*~ Unknown*

Being in the fitness industry for over two decades, I have had the opportunity to test just about every vitamin and supplement product on the market. Some of them worked very well while others didn't work at all. I personally try to get my vitamin and minerals from natural foods. I do, however, supplement amino acids and herbs when I feel a deficiency.

My intent here is to first help you understand the roles that vitamins, minerals, and amino acids play in the health of the human system. Secondly, I will identify the functions of each nutrient and, finally, the recommended dosage, if needed. This information will help you determine if you need supplementation in addition to your food.

Vitamins are organic substances necessary for life. Vitamins are essential for the normal functioning of our bodies and, with a few exceptions, cannot be manufactured or synthesized by the body. They are necessary for our growth, vitality, and general well-being. Vitamins are found in all natural foods. We must obtain vitamins from these foods or from dietary supplements. Here are a few facts:

- Vitamins cannot replace foods; they have no caloric value of their own and cannot be assimilated without food.
- Vitamins are not substitutes for protein or any other nutrients such as minerals, fats, carbohydrates, or water.
- You cannot take vitamins, stop eating, and expect to be healthy. Vitamins are supplements in addition to your food source.
- Vitamins are components of our enzyme systems that act like spark plugs, energizing and regulating our metabolism.
- Foods that are heated and reheated are depleted of nutrients (vitamins).

## How Nutrients Work

- The body simplifies nutrients in order to utilize them.
- Nutrients basically work through digestion.
- An ordinary meal leaves the stomach in three to five hours
- Watery substances leave the stomach quite rapidly. Fats remain considerably longer.

- Virtually all absorption of nutrients occurs in the small intestine

The liver is the main storage organ for fat-soluble vitamins and is a powerful detoxifying organ, breaking down a variety of toxic molecules and rendering them harmless. It stores vitamins, such as A, D, and E, and digested carbohydrates as glycogen, which is released to sustain blood sugar levels.

The pancreas provides the most important enzymes. And here are some more facts…

- The pancreas secretes insulin, which accelerates the burning of sugar in the body.
- Insulin is secreted into the blood, not the digestive tract
- The larger part of the pancreas manufactures and secretes pancreatic juices, which contain some of the body's most important digestive enzymes. Lipases, which splits fats; proteases, which splits protein; and amylases which splits starches.

Now let's look at the specifics of each individual nutrient. First we will review vitamins and the specific roles of each.

1 gram (g) = 1,000 (mg) milligrams = 1,000.000 (mcg) micrograms = IU = International unit

## a) Vitamins

*Vitamin A (and Carotene):* Vitamin A is a fat-soluble vitamin that promotes the production of lysozymes (anti-infectious agents) in tears, saliva, and sweat. Vitamin A also directly strengthens the immune system by stimulating the all-important thymus gland. On the other hand, carotene was thought to be a precursor of vitamin A, but we now know it is much more. As a precursor, carotene is also converted to vitamin A by the body, but not all of it is converted to vitamin A. What remains is as important because carotene is a powerful antioxidant that also protects the lipid or fatty layer of the human cell. (Dosage: 10,000 IU vitamin A, 25,000 IU carotene.)

*B Vitamins*: Have you ever wondered why there are so many B vitamins and only one each of the others? The reason for this is that most of the vitamins were named during the first twenty to thirty years of this century. Scientist were moving into unknown territory, and their techniques and equipment were not as sophisticated as they are today. They believed that the nutritional effects of the B vitamins were caused by a single substance, which they called vitamin B. They then discovered that different substances were pulling off the same functions in the body. These were named B1, B2, B3, and so on. So it turns out that endless B vitamins were pulled out of a pool of only a few distinct compounds. Although B vitamins occur together in foods, overlap in others, and share many functions, they are chemically distinct. The importance here is that B vitamins and other water-soluble nutrients are not effectively stored in the body. Since water-soluble vitamins are regularly flushed out of the body, deficiencies are easily developed. Any factor that increases the flow of water through the body, such as stress, exertion, and illness, will also flush water-soluble nutrients out of the body faster.

*Thiamine (B1)*: Thiamine is considered to be the spark plug of the body's engine. An inadequate amount of thiamine alters the burning of sugar for energy, which causes a wide range of bodily functions to falter. This includes the proper function of the brain, muscles, nervous system, digestion, heart, lungs, and immune system. Consider B1 our energy spark.

Thiamine-rich foods: brewer's yeast, chickpeas, kidney (beef), kidney beans, liver (beef), navy beans, pork, rice bran, brown rice, salmon, soy beans, sunflower seeds, wheat germ, and whole grain flour. (Dosage: 25-80 mg per day.)

*Riboflavin (B2)*: Our cells need the correct oxygen/blood sugar mixture to operate efficiently. Riboflavin is the key cofactor in the biochemical circuit that provides that correct mixture. When there is a deficiency in riboflavin, the eyes, nerves, adrenal glands, skin, and mucous membranes can deteriorate. In addition, riboflavin helps us respond to stress more effectively. We look better, see better, and behave better when we have enough riboflavin.

The main dietary sources are dairy products and meat.

Riboflavin-rich foods: almonds, brewer's yeast, dairy products, chicken, kidney (beef), and wheat germ

*Vitamin B3 (Niacinamide):* Niacin is necessary for the cells to breathe and utilize nutrients. It is essential for the production of the brain's neurotransmitters and its use for carbohydrates for energy. Forty or more different biomechanical reactions require adequate niacin. Niacin widens the diameter of the blood vessels and increases blood flow. Severe deficiencies in niacin can cause diarrhea, dermatitis, and dementia. Niacin may also help prevent and relieve mild anxiety, fatigue, insomnia, depression, and other mental malfunctions.

Niacinamide-rich foods: beets, brewer's yeast, chicken, fish, peanuts, pork, salmon, sunflower seeds, turkey, and veal. (Dosage: 30-125 mg per day.)

*Vitamin B5 (Pantothenic Acid)*: This powerful vitamin and antioxidant plays a central role in the production of intercellular energy in the brain and is required to synthesize brain neurotransmitters, such as acetylcholine. It can also help to protect against the damage to arteries caused by dietary cholesterol.

Pantothenic acid-rich foods: blue cheese, corn, eggs, lentils, liver (beef), lobster, all meats, peanuts, peas, soybeans, sunflower seeds, wheat germ, and whole grain flour. (Dosage: 50-250 mg per day.)

*Vitamin B6 (Pyridoxine):* Pyridoxine is a key factor in the body's utilization of proteins, fats, and carbohydrates. Without it, the cells cannot produce energy. The body cannot grow or in any way maintain itself without this vitamin. It supports the nervous system, teeth, bones, and actually, the entire protein and collagen structure of the body. Pyridoxine has also been known to help relieve premenstrual swelling and acne. Sixty-six bananas contain about 50 milligrams of B6. The only way to ingest optimal amounts of B6 is through supplementation.

Pyridoxine-rich foods: avocados, bananas, bran, carrots, lentils, rice, salmon, shrimp, soybeans, sunflower seeds, tuna, wheat germ, and whole grain flour (Dosage: 25-80 mg per day.)

*Vitamin B12 (Cyanocobalamin):* Cobalamin appears to work alongside folic acid. The body's utilization of folic acid, DNA and RNA synthesis, and the nervous system all depend on cobalamin. The usual dietary sources of B12 are meats, milk and milk products, poultry, and seafood. (Dosage: 100-400 mcg per day.)

*Folic Acid*: Also called folate and similar to B12, folic acid is required for the synthesis of DNA. It also depends on B12 to be reutilized by the body. Folic acid is required for the conversion of toxic byproducts of ordinary protein metabolism to beneficial amino acids.

Folic acid-rich foods: barley, most beans, almost all fruits, chickpeas, green leafy vegetables, lentils, peas, brown rice, soy beans, sprouts, and wheat germ. (Dosage: 400-800 mcg per day.)

*Vitamin C*: Vitamin C is essential to the formation of collagen, which is the fundamental glue of the body. Collagen is a protein that supports bone, skin, teeth, cartilage, tendon, and connective tissue. Of all the know antioxidants found in the body, the most powerful is vitamin C. In addition, vitamin C supports our ability to withstand stress of all kinds, including temperature stress. But stress also depletes vitamin C. Vitamin C also boost the immune system, encourages healing, and supports fertility. It is safe, inexpensive, and provides one of the brain's most powerful defenses against free-radical damage. Most fruits and vegetable are rich in vitamin C, especially citrus fruits. (Dosage: 1000-3000 g per day.)

*Vitamin D*: Vitamin D is one of the vitamins that we can make ourselves. It is called the sunshine vitamin because the body makes its own when exposed to sufficient sunlight. Vitamin D also aids in the absorption of phosphorus and calcium from the intestine and determines the deposit of these minerals in bones and teeth. In addition, when we have sufficient amounts of vitamin D, we can prevent osteoporosis. During the winter months in areas of the world where there is little to no sunlight, a basic vitamin D supplement may be needed. Also note that that products such as fortified dairy are enriched with artificial D2, which may not be as effective. (Dosage: as directed, if needed.)

*Vitamin E*: Vitamin E is a fat-soluble vitamin that is also considered an antioxidant with a powerful ability to combat free-radical damage. It has also been shown to have anti-inflammatory properties and can help to reduce gum inflammation and tartar. Low-fat diets that do not include vitamin E-rich foods can make it very difficult to reach the required needs. Vitamin E is found in oils such as peanut, sunflower, cottonseed, and corn. Almonds, sunflower seeds, walnuts, wheat germ, and whole grain flour are also vitamin E-rich foods. (Dosage 400 IU.)

*Coenzyme Q10*: CoQ10 is a compound that takes various forms. It is found in humans and in most animals, and is classified as CoQ or coenzyme Q10. It possesses the properties of an antioxidant most like vitamins C and E. The main role is the production of energy in brain cells. It also acts as a cell membrane protector against free radicals. CoQ10 is classified as a non-vitamin nutrient, meaning that it cannot be obtained from one's diet or manufactured in the body. The richest sources of CoQ10 are polyunsaturated fats, such as soybean oil. Monounsaturated fats, such as olive oil, contain moderate amounts, and saturated fats, including those found in coconut oil, have none. Tuna, sardines, mackerel, beef, and chicken contain moderate amounts, as do some nuts, such as peanuts and walnuts. The main source in vegetables would be spinach. (Dosage: 10-90mg per day.)

*Vitamin P (Bioflavonoids)*: Also known as OPCs, bioflavonoids are not really vitamins. They do not seem to be essential in quite the same way as vitamins or minerals. When an essential vitamin or mineral is removed from the diet, specific deficiency symptoms eventually occur. This does not happen when bioflavonoids are removed from the diet. Bioflavonoids truly come into their own as supplements. The effects are seen in three ways: through the strengthening of small blood vessel walls, by fighting free-radical cells, and by regulating various key enzymes. The principle sources are yellow and orange citrus fruits (more in the skin), pine bark, and grape seed. The bioflavonoids that come from pine bark and grape seed are known as OPCs. OPCs are twenty times stronger than vitamin C and fifty times stronger than vitamin E. Another added benefit of OPCs is that they recycle vitamins C and E, allowing longer protection for the body. In addition, recent data indicates taking OPCs can improve skin elasticity. We can get the benefits of this antioxidant by having 4oz of red wine per day. (Dosage: 150mg per day.)

## b) Minerals

Minerals are components of body tissues and fluids that work in combination with enzymes, hormones, vitamins, and transport substances throughout the body.

Some are cofactors for enzymes; others activate molecules in metabolic pathways. Minerals participate in nerve transmission, muscle contraction, cell permeability, blood formation, acid base balance, fluid regulation, protein metabolism, and energy production.

Minerals play a role in basically all bodily functions. Minerals work either in combination with each other or as antagonist to each other.

Some minerals play the same role as vitamins, as cofactors in biochemical reactions. Others are used as structural components of the body. A few, such as calcium, play both roles.

## c) **Amino Acids**

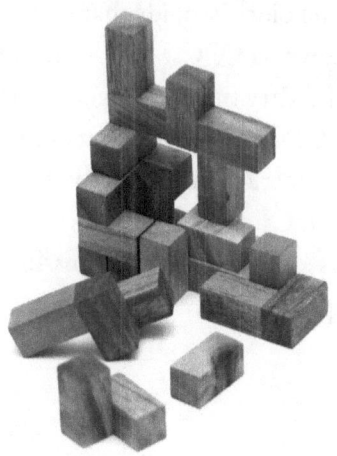

*Amino acids* are the basic building blocks of just about everything in the body. They are involved in making cells, repairing tissue, and helping the body fight infection. They build proteins and carry oxygen through the body. They come in two types:

*Nonessential* amino acids are the ones your body can manufacture from chemicals already in your system.

*Essential amino acids* can't be manufactured internally and have to be brought into the body via food or supplements.

Amino acids play a big role in repairing and rebuilding of cells in the brain and the body. And beyond vitamin- and mineral-type functions, amino acids are critical to the function of the brain and the communication of neurotransmitters. Amino acids can be found in almost all proteins, such as animal meats, fish, seafood, and eggs, as well as in smaller amounts in nuts and some soy products.

Our energy, or lack of energy, and moods are governed by the neurotransmitters in the brain. Amino acids help build and balance these neurotransmitters. A deficiency in the building blocks leads to imbalance in chemistry, and consequently leads to emotional instability. The following is a good example of how this works:

The neurotransmitter norepinephrine (aka, noradrenaline) provides us with both feelings of pleasure and motivation. It is derived from dopamine. Norepinephrine is involved in positive stress states, such as sex, being in love, music, dancing, and exercise. A deficiency in these neurotransmitters can lead to lack of motivation and drive, low self-esteem, and depression. If you crave stimulation from coffee, alcohol, sugar, or stress, you may be deficient. This is also called *reward deficiency syndrome* or (RDS). Those with RDS have a hard time feeling good or rewarded under normal conditions. Those with RDS can increase motivation and enhance moods by taking the precursor amino acids tyrosine and phenylalanine, also found in most proteins. These amino acids convert to dopamine with the help of the vitamins B6 and folic acid.

The following is a list of natural supplements and amino acids, how they work, and the positive and/or negative effects. This information will help you determine what supplementation you may need, if any. My personal belief is most foods are deficient or depleted of the raw nutrients. A perfectly balanced organic diet may give you all of the nutrients for optimum brain function, but missing one balanced meal can negatively change the chemical makeup of the brain and body. Remember, neurotransmitters are made from amino acids. Amino acids are the breakdown of proteins. Even a slight deficiency can lead to imbalance and emotional instability or MonkeyBrain! The following list is what I call super supplements. These are the nutrients that help keep the balance. In addition, these super supplements repair, rebuild, restore, and protect the body and the brain, including neurons and receptors in the brain.

# Super Supplements

## L Glutamine

- Dosage: 500 mg or 2-5 g per day (between meals)
- How it works: provides fuel for the brain and helps build and balance neurotransmitters
- Positive effects of supplementation: improves both mental energy and relaxation; reduces cravings, stabilizes blood sugar, and promotes memory
- *Cautions: rare reports of headaches at high doses*

## L Tyrosine

- Dosage:1000 mg, 1-2 times per day (on an empty stomach)
- How it works: tyrosine is a precursor to the neurotransmitter dopamine, adrenaline, noradrenaline, and the thyroid hormone, thyroxine
- Positive effects of supplementation: promotes energy and motivation, enhances mood, and supports healthy thyroid function
- Tyrosine-rich foods, such as lean red meat, chicken, and most animal meats, all provide sufficient amounts of the amino acid tyrosine, therefore it is beneficial to include these foods into each meal
- *Cautions: not recommended for those with a history of mania, unless under doctors care; should not be taken by people that are pregnant or nursing, people with phenylketonuria, or melanomas*

### DL Phenylalmine (DLPA)

- Dosage: 500 mg 1-2 times per day (on empty stomach)
- How it works: precursor for tyrosine, which converts to dopamine, adrenaline, and noradrenaline
- Positive effects of supplementation: promotes energy, controls appetite, relieves pain, and enhances mood
- *Cautions: not recommended for those with mental disorders, mania, or the metabolic disease phenylketonuria.*

### Omega 3

- Dosage: 500-1000 mg, 1-3 times per day (with meals), or eat fatty fish three times per week
- How it works: in addition to the health benefits it turns out it builds material for neuron membranes; enhances neural transmission, and increases serotonin levels
- Positive effects: improves learning, memory, and mood in depression
- Cautions: none

## Mood Enhancers

### 5-hydroxytryptophan (5-HTP)

- Dosage: for daytime use, 50-100 mg, 2-3 times per day. For sleep aid, 50-200 mg, one hour before bedtime. Also take about 50 mg of vitamin B6 as a cofactor.
- Like L-tryptophan, it is converted into serotonin, elevating mood, inducing relaxation, and improving sleep. 5-HTP is a direct precursor of serotonin and also enters the brain more easily than tryptophan. In addition, unlike

tryptophan, it can be taken with food or other amino acids with no interference. However, it still needs vitamin B6 as a cofactor for conversion to serotonin.

- How it works: as a direct precursor with vitamin B6 for the neurotransmitter serotonin
- Positive effects: suppresses appetite and promotes emotional stability, dreaming, and creativity; and, as mentioned before, it induces relaxation, elevates mood, and improves sleep.
- *Cautions: Some individuals have reported nausea and agitation at high doses. Should normal doses cause anxiety, in which case it should be stopped. Do not take 5-HTP with SSRI antidepressants except under medical guidance.*

## L-Tryptophan

- Dosage: 500-1000 mg, 2-3 times per day for depression and for insomnia. Take the dose one hour before bedtime.
- As cofactors, take 50 mg of vitamin B6, and a minimum of 15 mg of zinc. L-tryptophan is best absorbed with a carbohydrate snack.
- How it works: as a precursor of serotonin.
- Positive effects: promotes healthy sleep/wake patterns, deep sleep, dreaming, and creative imagination. And like 5-HTP, it elevates mood and promotes relaxation and emotional stability.
- *Cautions: In high doses, can cause nausea, headaches, constipation, and other gastrointestinal problems in certain people. It should not be taken during pregnancy, with MAO-inhibitors, or in cases of autoimmune disease Lupus. Do not take L-tryptophan or melatonin and SSRI antidepressants except under medical guidance.*

## St. John's Wort

- Dosage: Begin with 2 doses of 300 mg per day with food. If there is no change in mood after one week, increase to 300 mg, 3 times per day, or 2 doses of 450 mg per day, for a total of 900 mg.
- How it works: appears to inhibit reuptake of the neurotransmitter serotonin, noradrenaline, and dopamine, and enhances GABA activity as well.
- Positive effects: acts as an antidepressant, helps reduce anxiety in most people, and helps regulate sleep.
- *Cautions: St. John's Wort has not been researched sufficiently to recommend for use during pregnancy or nursing. May cause allergic reactions, rashes, and sun sensitivity in susceptible individuals. Can reduce the potency of protease inhibitors (taken as treatment for AIDS) or cycloporin (a rare immunosuppressant taken by organ transplant patients). In very few cases, has been shown to reduce the potency of birth control pills.*

## S-adenosyl-methionine (SAMe)

- Dosage: 200mg, 1-2 times per day, between meals
- How it works: Placebo-controlled, double-blind studies show that SAMe is equal or superior to antidepressants and most often works within a few days with no significant side effects. Instead, SAMe has side effects as an effective treatment for joint disease, fibromyalgia, and liver problems. SAMe is naturally occurring molecules, essential in the manufacture of neurotransmitters.
- Positive effects: improved learning, memory, and mood in depression, bipolar disorder, and dyslexia.
- Cautions: None

## Memory Boosters

### Ginkgo Biloba

- *Dosage*: 60-120 mg per day, 2 times per day.
- Ginkgo is an herbal remedy that has been used in the East for thousands of years for memory enhancement. Research has shown that ginkgo improves short-term and age-related memory loss. It is also known to improve circulation and poor blood flow to the brain. Ginkgo's healing properties appear to come from the chemicals known as flavonoids and terpene lactones. These powerful antioxidants help vitamin E and other antioxidants protect the brain from damage as well as aid in the production of neurotransmitters. They help to normalize acetylcholine receptors.
- How it works: improves circulation and act as an antioxidant
- Positive effects: improves cognitive performance
- Cautions: None reported

### DMAE

- Dosage: 100-300 mg daily, taken in the morning or midday, not in the evening. DMAE can take 2-3 weeks to work.
- DMAE crosses the blood-brain barrier and gets into the brain cells more rapidly. It accelerates the production of acetylcholine, reducing anxiety and racing minds. It improves concentration and learning.
- How it works: precursor for choline and crosses easily into the brain, helping to make acetylcholine. In higher doses, can act as a stimulant by enhancing dopamine activity.
- Positive effects: improves concentration, increases alertness, improves attention span, and normalizes brain wave patterns.

- *Cautions: Can cause overstimulation in higher doses and not recommended for those diagnosed with schizophrenia, mania, or epilepsy. Reduce the dose if you experience insomnia.*

## Acetyl-L-carnitine (ALC)

- Dosage: 250-1,500 mg daily, between meals.
- The amino acid carnitine can be used directly as a stimulant for the brain. It also acts as an antioxidant that protects against brain damage and keeps the nervous system healthy. ALC also helps to stimulate the growth of new brain cells and improves communication between the right and left hemispheres of the brain.
- How it works: acts as fuel for the brain, helps make acetylcholine, and acts as an anti-oxidant
- Positive effects: improves mood and mental performance
- *Cautions: not recommended for those with diabetes, liver or kidney disease*

In conclusion, here is what we do know:

- Vitamins are organic structures necessary for life and for the normal functioning of the brain and physical body.
- With the exception of a few, vitamins cannot be manufactured or synthesized by the body and must be obtained through our diet.
- The human body requires these things for optimum function:

1. Carbohydrates
2. Proteins
3. Fats
4. Water

- The nutrients that we receive from the carbohydrates, proteins, and fats are:

  1. Vitamins
  2. Minerals
  3. Amino Acids
  4. Water

- The three cornerstones to optimum mental, physical health, and performance are:

  1. Proper physical activity
  2. Balanced nutrition
  3. Sufficient sleep and rest

Now we can move on to the not-so-obvious things that affect our chemical balance and our emotions. It is time to smell the roses.

- Aromatherapy
*Nothing revives the past as completely as a*
*smell that was once associated with it.*
*~ Vladimir Nabokov*

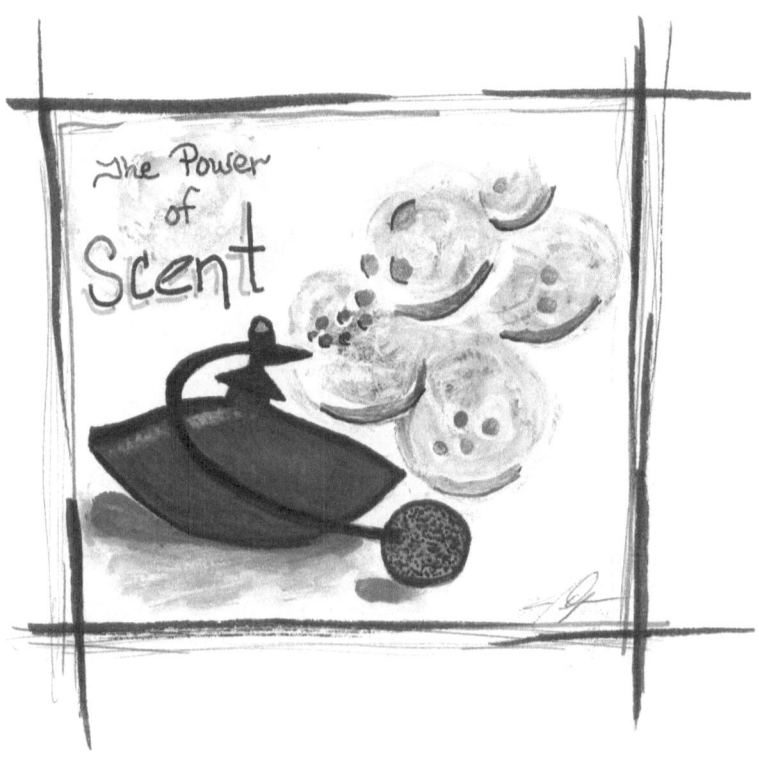

## The Power of Scent

Scent is the most basic of all senses and is vital for survival in the animal world, whether it be sniffing for danger, searching for food, or finding the perfect mate. Smells are carried directly by the olfactory nerves to the limbic system, a primitive part of the brain that acts like an emotional switchboard. The limbic system evaluates sensory stimuli—registering safety or danger, pleasure or pain—and directs our corresponding emotional responses: anger, fear, attraction, or repulsion. Because smell has the longest recall of all senses, particular scents can help us retrieve specific memories that we may associate with that scent. For instance, the scent of pine, cloves, or apple cider could remind you of a holiday experience. Scents can be a direct pathway to memory and emotions. Certain scents can relieve pain, recall deep-seeded memories, and affect personality and behavior. The term *aromatherapy* was first coined in the early part of the twentieth century by the French chemist René-Maurice Gattefossé to describe the medicinal use of essential oils.

These oils are the vital essence of the plant. Just as in humans, these are chemical messengers that act throughout the plant in response to stress, including environmental conditions. These plant hormones have multiple purposes and can affect us as well, by inhaling the fragrance, applying them topically, or ingesting them. Using fragrances may turn out to be one of the fastest ways to stimulate chemistry.[27] "Smells act directly on the brain, like a drug," [28]says Dr Alan Hirsch, a neurologist, psychiatrist, and the director of the Smell and Taste Treatment and Research Center in Chicago. Aromatherapy is described as a treatment to "promote health and well-being" through massage, inhalation, baths, and compresses with creams and lotions. This suggests that fragrance can reduce stress, sedate or invigorate, provide pain relief, and stimulate sensory awareness.

Different scents can produce specific emotional states, which are communicated through various neurotransmitters. One

---

[27]   Hirsch, Chemical Senses, Smellandtaste.org/?action=about
[28]   Hirsch, Chemical Senses, Smelland taste.org/?action=about

way to measure this is to monitor certain brain waves with an electroencephalograph, or EEG, when the patient is smelling many different scents in real time. We know from brain-wave frequency studies that smelling lavender increases alpha waves, which are associated with relaxation. Different scents can be used to stimulate or to relax. The scents that have been proven to have the most sedative effects are (in the order of effectiveness for relaxation): *lavender, bergamot, sandalwood, lemon,* and *chamomile.* By using these scents during times of relaxation, you can develop a conditioned response wherein the body and the mind are trained to associate the smell with the relaxed state. This is precisely why spas and massage studios use aromatherapy. This puts you in a relaxed state even before the massage.

And just the opposite: long distance truck drivers and others whose jobs depend on staying alert can now sniff specific formulas that help them do so. Train conductors in Japan and Russia can use an *odorphone* developed by V. Krasnov, a Russian professor of biology and odorology. This little mechanical device releases hot whiffs of pine, cedar, seaweed, or mushrooms. These scents stimulate dopamine, which provides that boost of energy. Even some airlines have jumped onto the scent bandwagon. Virgin Atlantic Airlines developed kits that are available to passengers containing floral-scented bath oils to prevent jetlag. Below you will find scents in categories. These scents can be ingested in various ways, such as candles, bath and massage oils, or herbs, or in several combinations.

# Calming Scents—Stimulating Scents

## Calming Scents (Cooling)

The following scents have been known to induce relaxation:
Lavender
Bergamot
Marjoram
Sandalwood
Lemon
Chamomile
Rose

## Stimulating Scents (Warming)

The following scents tend to stimulate:
Clove
Cinnamon
Lemon
Ylang-ylang
Fennel
Angelica
Cardamom
Basil
Jasmine
Eucalyptus
Peppermint
Jasmine
Black Pepper

The following scents stimulate to a lesser degree:
Rose
Patchouli

The following scents are both relaxing and stimulating:
Ylang-ylang
Rose
Patchouli
Sandalwood
Jasmine
Vanilla
Musk

*Jasmine* and *ylang-ylang* are both stimulating and relaxing, but these scents also stimulate the pituitary gland to secrete endorphins, creating the feelings of bliss and increased self–awareness. This is why jasmine, ylang-ylang, cinnamon, and coriander are used as aphrodisiacs. Common sense might say these effects would cancel each other out, but they actually produce a very enjoyable mood. They help reduce stress and tension, which allows for more passion.

Scents have powerful psychological benefits and can be used in room settings with candles and essential oils. Another way to achieve the psychological benefits of aromas is by using scented bath and massage oils as well as incense. Even the sight and aroma of a fresh bouquet of flowers in your environment can make you feel better. Experiment with various scents and find which works best for your needs. Since scent is a powerful way to influence brain chemistry, it is a great tool for a little boost of energy or to calm down. It is just another tool to help keep us balanced—or should I say, make us *better*.

# CHAPTER 10

# Music

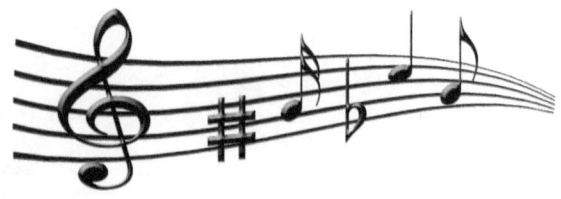

*Half an hour of music produces the same
effect as ten milligrams of Valium.*
*~ Raymond Bahr*

Music can be used as a powerful key to our bodies and psyches. For thousands of years, people throughout the world have used music to heal the mind, body, and spirit.

The field of sound healing has begun to emerge again into public awareness. Recent studies have shown that music can reduce stress, enhance the immune system, and slow down and even balance brain wave activity. The right music can even reduce muscle tension, increase endorphin levels, and trigger feelings of love and inner peace.

At the Addiction Research Center in Stanford, California[29], people listened to various kinds of music, including marching bands, spiritual anthems, and movie soundtracks. Almost half of the listeners reported feelings of euphoria, leading the

---

[29]   Ibid., 145

researchers to suspect that the joy of music is linked to the release of endorphins. To test the theory, the researchers injected the participants with naloxone, which blocks opiate (endorphin) receptors. Just as they expected, the listeners experienced far less pleasure. This suggests that certain types of music can actually boost endorphins.

There is also research on the effects of music on stress levels. Clinical psychologist and music therapist Mark Rider[30] tested cortisol levels on a dozen nurses under high stress.

You may recall reading about cortisol in Part I. Cortisol is secreted by the adrenal glands during the fight-or-flight stress response. When the nurses listened to soothing music and practiced relaxation, their rhythms were balanced and their stress hormones were reduced. Other days when the nurses did not listen to the music, their rhythms were out of balance and their hormones were significantly higher. Relaxation is not the only benefit of music. Upbeat music such as techno or rock & roll can increase energy levels and improve mood as well.

Music varies from Gregorian chants to heavy metal, and depending on your state of mind at the time, you can use music to calm you down or speed you up. It's all a matter of preference, and you can experiment with different types to fit your needs. Try all types of music. Pay attention to the way you feel when listening to the music. Are you more relaxed? Does it excite you and give you motivation? Does it make you sad? Does it make you happy?

---

30    Dr. Rider, Music Therapy, stress.org/music-therapy

For example, you may need an upbeat tempo in the morning to give you a little boost. On the other hand, the sounds of nature or soft rhythms in the evening could calm you down and help you sleep better. Here you can see how music can help us change mood and attitude, making us feel *better*.

# PART III

# *The Spirit*

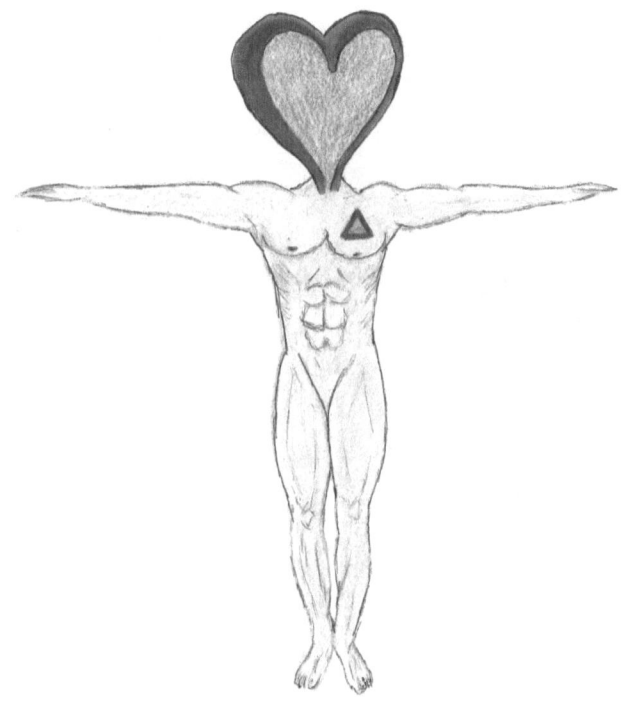

*All major religious and spiritual traditions carry basically the same message: that is love, compassion, and forgiveness. The important thing is they should be part of our daily lives.*
*~Dalai Lama*

In Part I, we looked at the brain and how MonkeyBrain and stress can make us sick. We also looked at ways to improve brain function. Part II explored various ways to improve our health, such as exercise, balanced nutrition, sufficient sleep, and better stress-coping skills.

Now, we will explore what can make us even better. First, we will define spirituality. Then we will look at the relationship between spirituality, health, and disease to see if there is a scientific connection. We are looking for the scientific nature of spirituality.

We will be addressing the spirit just as we did the brain and the body—scientifically first. Before we begin, let us look at a common meaning of spirituality. It includes activities that renew, lift up, comfort, heal, and inspire us and those with whom we interact. In other words, we are in spirit when we are good to ourselves and when we are good to those around us. This isn't about comparing one religion to another; this is about the health benefits of spiritual and religious practices.

In the early twentieth century, a doctor by the name of William James had a theory that religion influenced our health, particularly through the central nervous system. However, at that time and for many decades later, science became more focused on pragmatic research (relating to matters of fact), and the study of religion was left to the theologians.[31] At that time, scientists were not studying the health benefits of spiritual and religious practices.

However, more recently there has been resurgence in the scientific understanding of what spirituality is and how it influences our health. The science indicates that, in general, overall mortality

---

[31]   Wang, *The Neuroscience of Everyday Life*, www.thegreatcourses.com.

and longer life expectancy were found to be more common in religious or spiritual people.[32] Now the question is: Why? Are spiritual and religious individuals healthier and happier because of behavior? The answer is yes, behavior does play a role in our health.

For example, Utah has a lower rate of cardiopulmonary disease. This is partly due to a large population of Mormons who live there. Mormons, for the most part, do not smoke. So in this case, the reasoning for better health in this population is behavior. Also this population tends to practice other behavior, such as prayer and meditation. So which is it?

Well, we know for sure that smoking contributes to many diseases, but does prayer and meditation make us healthier? The answer is yes! The latest research indicates the practice of prayer and meditation has positive benefits on cardiovascular health. In addition, there is promising data in the area of the nervous system, specifically the activation of the parasympathetic nervous system.[33] You may recall the review on the autonomic nervous system in Part I. The PNS lowers the heart rate, lowers blood pressure, lowers respiratory rate, and increases digestion.[34] So we can see why anything that activates the PNS makes us better. The physiological effects are obvious: better cardiovascular health, better stress response, and better digestion.

What this indicates is the practice of prayer or meditation activates the system that brings us down and deactivates the system that brings us up. In other words, these disciplines reduce and possibly

---

[32]  Satterfield, Mind-Body Medicine, www.thegreatcourses.com.

[33]  Satterfield, Mind-Body Medicine. www.thegreatcourses.com.

[34]  Satterfield, Mind-Body Medicine, www.thegreatcourses.com.

inhibit the release of stress hormones while triggering the release of feel-good chemicals, such as serotonin, GABA, and oxytocin.

The spiritualty and health research also looked at some other common traditions that are considered spiritual or religious practices, such as acceptance, forgiveness, compassion, gratitude, and acts of service, and the relation between illness and disease.[35]

> *"If you want others to be happy, practice compassion.*
> *If you want to be happy, practice compassion."*
> ~ *Dalai Lama*

The data indicates positive health benefits from all of these practices. Let us look at forgiveness in particular. Forgiveness is very much related to acceptance. There are actually a number of studies that looked at the health effects of forgiveness. Many of these studies remind us that forgiveness is not about forgetting or resignation. Forgiveness and reconciliation are different. Forgiveness is an active and ongoing process that might actually take years to evolve. The primary beneficiary of forgiveness is the person doing the forgiving. The person who has wronged you may no longer be in your life or even alive. You are the one who benefits, particularly from a cardiovascular perspective.[36] Interestingly, all of these practices activate the parasympathetic nervous system, triggering the release of oxytocin and lowering the heart rate. Again, we are talking about not what makes us well, but what we can do to make us better. Therefore, forgiveness is a sure way to make us better. After looking at the research and data on forgiveness, I wanted to test it myself. I decided to forgive someone in my personal life that I felt had betrayed me.

---

[35]   Satterfield, Mind-Body Medicine, www.thegreatcourses.com.
[36]   Satterfield, Mind-Body Medicine, www.thegreatcourses.com.

At this time, I still engaged my thoughts with bad memories that enflamed the emotions of resentment and anger often. The MonkeyBrain was out in full force. I was looking for revenge. I knew that these emotions were not good for my physical or emotional health because I could feel my blood boil by merely thinking of that person.

Remember, the increase in epinephrine (adrenaline) and cortisol increase the heart rate as our warning. If we don't acknowledge the cause of the blood boil, we cannot bring it back down. Whatever is causing the blood to boil is the thing that needs healing. If you look at this from a chemical perspective, the chemicals driven by the sympathetic nervous system (warming) increase the heart rate and cause the boiling feeling. The chemicals driven by the parasympathetic nervous system (cooling) lower the heart rate. In other words, in order to reduce the SNS warming chemicals, we have to activate the PNS with the cooling chemicals. This requires action and activity in that direction. I knew, chemically speaking, that the feelings of love and compassion activated the PNS, which resulted in reducing the activity of the SNS and the warming chemicals that were causing my blood to boil.

I then tried a little experiment. I wanted to see if my memories of the love I had for this person in the past would help me reduce the anger that I felt at the time. I call this story *The Magical Love Letter*. I began to think of all of the good things and good times with this person. I pulled every good memory of this person that I could think of and started writing them down, one by one. By the time I had reached the bottom of the paper, I noticed a shift. The boil was gone! As I was writing down all of those good memories, my brain began to release cooling chemicals that eventually activated the PNS, and at the same time deactivated the SNS, essentially inhibiting the release of adrenaline and cortisol (the boil). It allowed the cooling chemicals to override the warming ones. I realized at that moment what had happened. The chemicals oxytocin, also known as the *moral molecule*, and vasopressin trumped adrenaline and cortisol! This proved to me that if given a chance, love and compassion override hate and resentment. It was a pivotal moment in my own self-awareness. I learned that forgiveness is an ongoing process and we can accelerate that process by changing the way that we feel about whatever the situation is that is causing the boil. The process may require using numerous ways to forgive. *The Magical Love Letter* is a great tool in the process of forgiveness.

> *"Holding on to anger is like grasping a hot coal*
> *with the intent of throwing it at someone else;*
> *but you are the one who gets burned."*
> *~ Buddha*

In addition, studies indicate that practices such as forgiveness, gratitude, and acceptance have been predictors of positive emotion. This includes spiritualty and religiosity.[37] It seems that belonging to a religious or spiritual group or community has a direct correlation to our health as a whole. Studies have been done on groups of people who gather together for the same religious or spiritual purpose with a common bond, and these people tend to have lower levels of stress hormones and better overall health, including better emotional health.[38]

There are several reasons for this. First, we know the biological and neurological health benefits are significant. These benefits include improved resting heart rate, improved blood pressure,

---

[37]    Satterfield, Mind-Body Medicine, www.thegreatcourses.com.
[38]    Satterfield, Mind-Body Medicine, www.thegreatcourses.com.

and improved cardiovascular reactivity (lower stress response and faster recovery).

But more importantly are the positive effects that these practices have on our chemical balance and emotional stability. Therefore, it does make sense that those who practice spirituality will have better overall health. Regardless of how and why these practices became the pillars of religion and spiritual traditions, they trigger the release of chemicals that activate the parasympathetic nervous system. To be more specific, these activities trigger the release of the chemical oxytocin and vasopressin, among many others. We know that these chemicals can inhibit the release of stress hormones, such as epinephrine aka/adrenaline and cortisol. These practices also trigger the release of rewarding feel-good chemicals, such as serotonin, GABA, and even endorphins, all of which enhance our mood. So do we feel better in church or in spiritual groups because of bonding and the release of oxytocin and other feel-good chemicals? Or is it something higher? I will leave it up to you to answer that question.

For me, however, this question made me look at spiritualty from a chemical point of view. I did this without the use of a church or group setting. I began to test this theory by doing some of the things that were considered religious practices or spiritual development. I added a daily practice of gratitude and yoga in addition to my physical conditioning workout. I didn't necessarily exclude organized religion, but I did open my mind to all theories, religious and spiritual, as well as the biological and chemical. What I noticed were positive changes in my stress response, my behavior, and my attitude. We now know what activities trigger a cascade of chemicals that have a profound positive effect on our health. Therefore, I concluded that we could condition the spirit just as we can train the brain and strengthen the physical body.

Although the brain, body, and the spirit are interdependent, the activities that strengthen each are different. And since oxytocin is the one chemical that has the ability to reduce and/or inhibit the release of stress hormones,[39] why not practice those things that trigger the release of this chemical?

So it doesn't matter how spiritual or religious we are; our thoughts and emotions are driven by chemicals. These chemicals are stimulated by our behavior—all of it. As I mentioned earlier, we are essentially designed biologically and chemically to feel good if we do good for ourselves and when we are good to others. On the other hand, we feel bad when we are not so good to ourselves or not good to others. With the exception of the seriously mentally ill, we are all hardwired in this way.

> *"The human spirit is stronger than anything that can happen to it."* ~ CC Scott

The bottom line is this: spirituality is within us all. And that spirit within us is influenced and strengthened with specific behavior that has been discussed throughout this book. If you do things to raise your heart rate, you should also counter those things with activity that lowers the heart rate. Many spiritual practices lower the heart rate, therefore putting them in the category of what we can do to make us better.

Trying to define spiritualty in words was a challenge for me. I think it is best expressed in feelings. It is the feelings that we get when we do good. For example, I returned from shopping and noticed that I wasn't charged for an item that was in the bag. I then contemplated whether or not I should go back and pay for the item. The next

---

[39]    Wang, The Neuroscience of Everyday Life, www.thegreatcourses.com.

thoughts were completely ego-driven. I began to think about how many times I may have been overcharged. It was followed by, *I'm too tired. I'll pay them back the next time I shop there.* These contemplations went back and forth. But I finally asked myself, "What is the right thing to do?" The answer was very obvious. I returned to the store and paid the money that was owed. On the way home, I felt very good and realized the action that I took in this case triggered the release of a cascade of feel-good chemicals, similar to the spiritual work mentioned earlier. What I'm trying to say is: We are practicing spiritualty when we do what we feel is right. It's the feeling we get when we help another in need, when we have compassion, when we are creating or learning. We are in spirit when we are in awe of a beautiful sunset or observing wildlife in its raw form. Spirituality surrounds us, and if we look for it, we will always find it. My conclusion was that spiritualty was not about an organization or anything outside of ourselves, although it can't hurt! Spiritualty is within us all. Being spiritual is a behavior that makes us better, and this behavior is strengthened when we do good for ourselves and for others. This is partly because we have a specific mass of oxytocin receptors in the brain, heart, and throughout the body. Oxytocin is the one chemical that essentially makes us feel good by doing good. I didn't learn this by studying spiritualty or brain chemistry. I learned this by practicing the attitude of gratitude, practicing acceptance and forgiveness, and being compassionate and kind while serving others. What I learned as I introduced these practices into my daily life was that I felt better. And it turns out, my energy rubbed off on every other person that I encountered.

> *"What we see depends mainly on what we are looking for."*
> *~ John Lubbock*

Earlier we talked about what makes us sick and what makes us well. Here we are looking at what makes us better. What I mean by better is: better cardiovascular health and improved function of the nervous system.[40] Again, here we are talking about the health benefits of spirituality. It just so happens that things such as *prayer, mediation, gratitude, trust, compassion,* and *acceptance* have been spiritual practices for hundreds, if not thousands, of years. We don't have to be part of any organization to benefit from practicing these things; we just have to practice them.

The energy that we radiate out to others is determined by how we feel. How we feel is determined by what we do, all of it! Everything that we see, hear, taste, touch, or smell and all emotionally charged thoughts stimulate some neurotransmitter that makes us feel good or not so good. This feeling then radiates from us and is felt by every person that we encounter. I'm not trying to use the labels good or bad, but we all know when we do things that just aren't right. With that said, here is my opinion about spirituality: Some of us can be deeply spiritual, yet not be religious. I believe that the spirit is energy, and that energy is everywhere. We are spiritual beings living in human bodies, but it doesn't matter how spiritual we are. If our human body and brain are not healthy and balanced, neither is the spirit.

Spiritual development is a process, and it is best achieved with a healthy brain/mind and body. The process and path is different for everyone, but we are here on this earth to expand in all ways: physically, mentally, and spiritually. We are here to learn and grow with each experience and to share that growth with others. The purpose of life is to prosper, to love, to live it, to be the best that we can be—to reach out without fear for new experiences and create a life with purpose. And remember, spiritual awareness is connected to physical and mental health. This is the brain, body,

---

[40]    Satterfield, Mind-Body Medicine, www.thegreatcourses.com.

and spirit connection. Spiritual development requires committed action over time. Just like the brain and the body, when you do the work, the reward follows. When you stop doing the work, the results are diminished.

> *"We either make ourselves miserable or we make ourselves strong. The amount of work is the same."*
> ~ *Carlos Castaneda*

Now let us move on to the practical work and integrate the *stuff* that makes us better. The next few chapters will look at some of the behavior that makes us better.

# Spiritual Development

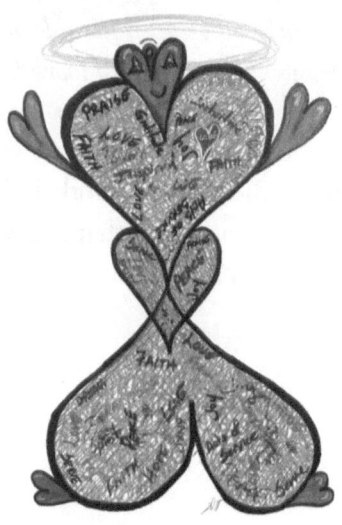

*Nothing ever goes away until it has taught us what we need*
*to learn. The lessons that we learn strengthen the spirit.*
*~ Richard Carlson*

Now that we know a little more about the effects of spirituality on our health and emotions, we can introduce some of the work. The following sections include some of the practices that have been religious and spiritual traditions for thousands of years. Just remember this isn't about comparing one religion or spiritual practice to another; it is about behavior that improves our health and makes us better.

We basically know what makes us sick: poor nutrition, lack of movement, not enough sleep, stress, pollution, and unhealthy behavior. We also know what makes us well: balanced nutrition, proper exercise, sufficient sleep, low stress levels, and a healthy environment. Now we will explore the things that make us healthier, or should I say *better!* Let's explore some specific behavior and practices, such as mindfulness, balance work, gratitude, love, and positive thinking.

The research indicates that all of these practices have significant health benefits, especially in the area of cardiovascular health, emotional health, and the nervous system.[41] It doesn't matter what we call it; just know that these practices improve the entire human system.

## a) Mindful Training

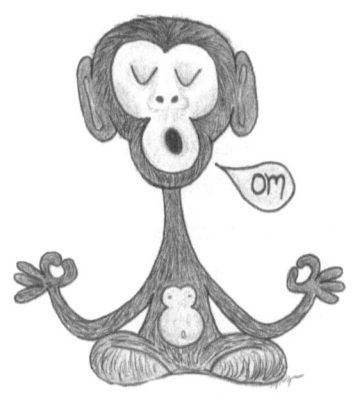

*"The best way to cage the monkey is to silence the brain."*

Here we are going explore the benefits of meditation, or what I consider mindful training. We are most familiar with meditation through Eastern religions. However, Judaism, Islam, and

---

[41]   Satterfield, Mind-Body Medicine, www.thegreatcourses.com.

Christianity have meditation traditions as well. Most meditation techniques involve focusing on one thing, such as the breath, a mantra, or a specific object or symbol. This practice is usually done for ten to twenty minutes.

The brain is ordinarily bombarded with stimulation, such as thought processes, hunger, fear, or pain. By focusing on a specific thing, the brain begins to quiet down.[42] There are many different forms of meditation; including movement meditation, such as walking and focusing on the breath. Meditation is really just about allowing the mind to become still. It is about being mindful of the brain's activity and allowing the brain (the engine), to rest.

> *"We need quiet time to examine our lives openly and honestly … spending quiet time alone gives your mind an opportunity to renew itself and create order."*
> *~ Susan L. Taylor*

With time and practice, you will find that quieting your brain and body on a regular basis will allow you to reach an elevated state of awareness. In this elevated state of awareness, the physical body relaxes and emotions settle down. This state of mind is real, and it correlates to distinctive changes in brain wave patterns. The four wave patterns are beta, alpha, delta, and theta. Beta waves are highly active waves that dominate when we are awake. Alpha waves are slower rhythms. Delta waves are our sleep state, and theta wave rhythms are in between waking and sleep. Theta wave rhythms are predominant during light sleep or extreme relaxation, as well as meditation and even activities such as yoga and tai chi.[43]

---

[42]  Satterfield, Mind-Body Medicine, www.thegreatcourses.com.
[43]  Johnson, Brain Wave Research, www.brainwave-research-institute.com/

Most of what we do every day is speed up. We rarely slow down, with the exception of sleep.

> *"Meditation takes place when you bring all of your awareness to the moments. Forget the past and the future, and observe the present as it comes. This is mindful living."*

Take a good look at your daily activities, your behavior, and your habits. If most are on the hot side, meaning dopamine-driven, begin to incorporate cool activities to bring yourself back to balance. You may refer back to Chapter 2; there you can see the list of activities and behaviors: warming ones that raise the heart rate, and cooling ones that bring the heart rate back down. Mindful meditation, yoga, and tai chi are very effective at bringing the heart rate down.

For me, it was very hard to quiet my brain enough to reach a meditative state, so I tried many different techniques and at different times of the day. I found myself still struggling to quiet my thoughts. As a matter of fact, the harder I tried, the less relaxed I became. One day, when I didn't have time to do all my work, I decided to do all of my conditioning in one session. I did my strength training first, followed by yoga and balance exercises. I then set the timer for ten minutes and sat down to meditate.

For the first time, I was able to quiet my thoughts within a few deep breaths. The next thing that I was aware of was the buzzer on the timer going off. I felt so good that I set the timer for another ten minutes and went back to my breathing. Again I was able to totally relax and didn't move until the buzzer went off. Immediately I realized why there was a dramatic change in my ability to relax. It was chemical. By doing the exercising first, I changed the chemical makeup of my brain, which allowed me to reach a meditative state much sooner.

Remember, exercise reduces mental and physical tension, and yoga takes it to another level by activating the parasympathetic nervous system and lowering the heart rate. This is when I realized that I needed to influence my brain chemistry using movement to activate the cooling chemicals. In other words, I first needed to workout intensely to reduce the adrenaline and cortisol. This then allowed for the release of acetylcholine, serotonin, endorphins, and GABA. Now the yoga, balance work, and meditation triggered the release of oxytocin and others that we may not be aware of yet, activating the parasympathetic nervous system. You may recall in Chapter 2 the review on neurotransmitters and hormones, where the cooling chemicals are necessary for relaxing the brain and the physical body. My experiment, combining and integrating several disciplines, resulted in a brain/body conditioning program that, if done properly and consistently, produces improvement in all areas: brain, body, and spirit.

The Joyefit Fusion is structured to create the perfect chemical makeup for meditation or even just relaxing. For me, meditation is not about a specific position or mantra but more about just releasing tension and reducing the brain chatter. I prefer to lay flat on my back with my head propped up, but I do use the seated position as well. Position is more of a personal preference. It is, however, very important to breathe full, deep breaths. What is important is that you take full diaphragmatic breaths, inhaling and filling the diaphragm first and then the lungs, followed by a full exhalation. I have found it beneficial to count four seconds on the inhale and six seconds on the exhale. Once you have trained yourself to breathe deeply, the count is not necessary.

Meditation takes time, patience, and commitment. I find it helpful to use a timer. Begin with five minutes and work up to twenty minutes when possible. If you are anything like me, it will take some time to slow your brain's thinking. After all, thinking is what the brain does. Just allow the thoughts to come and go. Do not engage in the thoughts, especially if the thoughts are of things that you do not want. Just bring your attention back to your breath. We actually can't think and take a full deep breath at the same time, making it the best way to get out of your thoughts. I do recommend calming music, preferably without lyrics. Remember, the brain will associate words in the songs with your personal experiences, and that alone will trigger the brain to think more. Before you say, I can't, think, I can try. The brain will take the instructions and act accordingly, which is, I can.

The goal is to breathe and shrink or temporarily eliminate the brain chatter. *Cage the monkey!* Just breathe and relax the entire body and release the tension. The most important part of this program is the order in which it is done. Remember, it is about activating the right chemicals at the right time. It is about reducing the activity of the sympathetic nervous system while activating the parasympathetic nervous system and lowering the heart rate. Mindful training, such as meditation, is a sure way to make us better. The benefits will be gratifying, and once it becomes a habit, you will crave this quiet time.

## b) Goals—Intentions

*"Setting a small realistic goal is the first step in turning the invisible into the visible."~ Unknown*

Setting goals or intentions is very effective for helping you achieve, accomplish, create, or receive a desired outcome. Part II explained a strategy known as SMART goals.[44] This goal strategy is designed to make the goals clear: specific, measurable, action-oriented, realistic, and timely. Personal and professional change requires a plan of action. Setting goals this way is essentially your detailed plan of action. Set short-term goals that lead to the ultimate outcome. At this point, you should have logged your physical body improvement SMART goals. You can now implement the actions into the twenty-one-day challenge. Now you can add to your physical body goals with brain and spiritual smart goals.

Our focus for the twenty-one-day challenge is to improve in the areas of brain, body, and spirit. Setting goals in each area of life will help ensure balance and continued growth. In addition to setting goals to improve physical, mental, and spiritual health it is also important to look at the following areas of your life:

- Family
- Home
- Career and financial
- Friendships
- Culture and education
- Recreation and leisure

You can set goals in all areas. The objective is to have a detailed plan of action. This allows your brain to focus on the details, and then the brain and the mind will look for ways to help you accomplish those things. It is like giving the brain and the mind detailed instructions to follow. It is a way to make the brain and the mind work with you, not against you. Review the goals that you have already set in Part II and make sure that they are

---

[44] Gavin, Lifestyle Fitness Coaching, 168.

specific, realistic, and clear as well as consistent with your abilities and values.

*"Our intention creates our reality."*
~ *Wayne Dyer*

Now let us talk a bit about intentions. Intentions are extensions of the goals. Here is where you extend the goal with more detail and express it in the future. Intentions are written as if the goals have already been accomplished.

We will use the example given in Part II. The goals were to improve physical, mental, and spiritual health, lose weight, learn something new, begin a gratitude journal, and so on. Setting intentions for these goals is like writing the story after the fact.

For example, "I feel and look so good since I lost those few pounds. I love being able to fit into my favorite jeans. My attitude is so much better since I started practicing gratitude and my friends have started calling to hang out again. Learning how to play golf has been so fun and challenging, plus I've met some great new friends."

With intentions, you are giving the subconscious, detailed instructions with emotional attachment to begin the manifestation process. Remember, the mind is always there to help you make things happen, but you have to give it clear instructions. When writing goals or intentions, avoid statements like, "I *will* lose weight" or "I *don't* want to be alone." Instead use statements like "I *have* my ideal body" or "I *attract* the perfect partner who loves me the way I am." Always write your intentions like a story and try to evoke emotion as if you have already achieved the outcome. The more detail that you put into the statement, the more accurate the outcome becomes. Intentions are basically prayers in writing.

> *"For things to change, we must change. For*
> *things to get better, we must get better."*
> *~ Heidi Wills*

In other words, believe it will happen and you will find a way to make it happen. The story in Chapter 1, *MonkeyBrain in the Airplane,* is a great example of writing intentions of the best-case scenario. You may recall I used the intentional shifting technique to fake my brain into believing my feel-good statements. At the time, my goal was to reduce my stress levels, but my brain took the statements as truth and consequently changed a bad situation into the best possible outcome.

The objective with this exercise is to be clear about your desires. It doesn't matter how you make your desires heard; just make sure that your head is void of other thoughts and be clear. Also make sure your goals and intentions are consistent with your values.

Don't be afraid to set high goals, so long as they are realistic. Remember, one goal leads to another, and another, and so on. If your goal is to be a musician, by all means, set your intentions and then begin the process of learning the trade. You have to know how to play a musical instrument before you become a rock star. Make your intentions clear and then write down how (what actions you will take) and when (give yourself a time frame or deadline) you will achieve the goal. When we do the work, the reward always follows. Remain patient, consistent, and focused, and the reward will follow. You are in the process of improving your life one day at a time.

Share what you have learned and help others with the process. Once we know better, we should do better.

> *"You are never too old to set another goal*
> *or to dream another dream."*
> *~ C. S. Lewis*

## c) Spiritual Dance/Balance Work

This portion of the program is designed to create self-awareness and brain/body balance. Slow, methodical movement with balance helps regulate and balance brain chemistry in the emotional regions of the brain known as the amygdala and hypothalamus.[45] The balance work is a combination of breathing, slow movements with balance poses, and stretches, similar to yoga or tai chi. This program is beneficial for everyone, regardless of age, strength, or activity level. It is designed to improve focus, concentration, balance, and coordination, while improving strength and flexibility.

> *"Yoga is not about holding a perfect pose or being able to stand*
> *on your head. Balance work is a practice that doesn't judge*
> *perfection or imperfection. The health benefits are a result*
> *of practice with committed action over time. That is why it's*
> *called a practice. We must practice to receive the benefits."*
> *~ Unknown*

Integrate this work into your program as recommended in Part II. Most forms of yoga and tai chi will provide you with similar benefits.

---

[45]    Restak, Optimizing Brain Fitness, www.thegreatcourses.com

However, the advanced Joyefit Fusion workout DVD is very specific and structured. For additional instructions, motivation, inspiration, and continued support, you can purchase the DVD package at www.joyefit.com.

## d) Gratitude

> *"Be thankful for what you have; you'll end up having more. If you concentrate on what you don't have, you will never, ever have enough." ~ Oprah Winfrey*

Over the past decade, countless studies have indicated the social, physical, and psychological benefits of gratitude. The research suggests these benefits apply to anyone who practices gratitude, even during stress, illness, and disease. This includes elderly people confronting death, those with cancer, and people coping with other chronic diseases.[46]

Practicing gratitude has proven to be one of the most reliable methods for increasing satisfaction in life. Having gratitude increases the feelings of optimism, joy, enthusiasm, and other positive emotions. The positive health benefits include strengthened immune system, lower blood pressure, less aches and pains, and improved functioning of the nervous system.

If that isn't enough to convince you of the benefits of practicing gratitude, here are a few more:

- Gratitude promotes forgiveness.
- Gratitude reminds us to pay it forward. People who are grateful are more helpful and compassionate.

---

[46]    Miller, The Mental Health Benefits of Gratitude, www.intelihealth.com.

- Grateful people sleep well. Studies indicate that in general, they get more hours of sleep each night and spend less time awake before falling asleep. So instead of counting sheep to fall asleep, count your blessings.
- Gratitude also makes us more resilient. The studies found that those who are grateful recover from traumatic events, including war veterans with post-traumatic stress disorder.

So you can see, the benefits of practicing gratitude are overwhelming. Now the question is, how do we cultivate gratitude? Feeling grateful is a skill we can develop with practice. According to the latest research, here are some of the most effective ways to cultivate gratitude:[47]

- Begin by keeping a gratitude journal. Start by writing three to five things that you are grateful for every day.
- In addition, add why you are grateful for those things. For example, "I am so grateful for my family because their love and support makes my life better." Or, "I am so thankful for the bonus that I received from work because I now have the money for a vacation." (The twenty-one-day journal provides space so that you can begin to log your gratitude for each day.)

The practice of gratitude is also a very powerful way to stimulate rewarding and feel-good chemicals. When we are grateful and thankful for what we have *now*, we not only feel better, we also make those around us feel better. This is both chemical and spiritual in nature. Are you grateful for your loved ones? Are you grateful for your home, your transportation, or your job? Are you thankful for the wide variety of foods that keep you healthy and

---

[47]    Miller, The Mental Health Benefits of Gratitude, www.intelihealth.com.

alive or for the utility companies that supply you with fresh water and energy that make your life better? In today's busy society, we tend to expect things and forget all of the small things that make our lives better, such as an abundance of food and clean drinking water. There are millions of people around the world who do not have these things. I am often reminded of the Hindu expression:

*"A man who has no shoes is glad he has feet."*

I had to train myself to be grateful. I really didn't feel the positive chemical shift in my body from the feelings of gratitude until I began to write a gratitude journal. The list made me more aware of the things that I was grateful for in real time, and those things became everything in life. This practice has a powerful effect on our mind/body balance. You don't have to take my word for it; try it yourself. For the next twenty-one days, just three weeks, write down three to five things that you are grateful for and why. It doesn't matter what you are grateful for, just start being grateful and watch what happens. Use the twenty-one-day journal to document your gratitude, and pay attention to your feelings when practicing this discipline. Consider the gratitude journal a part of your spiritual exercises. Gratitude is probably the most important thing that we can do to make us happy. Therefore, gratitude is a sure way to make us better!

# CHAPTER 12

# The Power of Thought

*"A positive mind finds a way it can be done. A*
*negative looks for all the ways it can't be done."*
~ Napoleon Hill

The power of positive thought, in my opinion, is the most important change you can make in your life. Let me begin by reminding you that that the brain, in most of us, is in the cognitive unconscious up to 80 percent of the time, which means our thoughts are out of our conscious control much of the time, good or bad. That is something to keep in mind while reading this information.

Most of our suffering is not from what happens to us, but how we think about what happens to us. And this is not just about thought. It is more about the chemistry and energy that is created by the thought. This is known as the *law of attraction*. It is defined as how we attract, by some mysterious way, people, things, circumstances, and situations that appeal either in a negative or positive way that correspond to our emotions and energy. This is human energy, or as it is called in physics, *quantum mechanics*. A quantum is a unit of energy, and mechanics is the movement of energy. In the brain, this happens from one cell to another. To be more specific: the energy travels from the (electric/energy) pre synaptic neuron to the (chemical) post-synaptic neuron, which stimulates the chemicals that create the way we feel. The emotion triggered by these chemicals determines the energy that others around us feel. How many times have you met someone and said,

"I felt that man didn't like me," or "That lady had great energy." This is human energy.

> *"The game of life is a game of boomerang. Our*
> *thoughts, deeds, and words return to us sooner*
> *or later with astounding accuracy."*
> ~ *Florence Scovel Shinn*

Thought energy is nothing new. Albert Einstein discovered this long ago, but his theory was discredited for many years. However, he has since been proven correct once again. The law of quantum physics is now the law of physics, just as the law of gravity is a part of physics as well. And quantum mechanics is just as relevant to the brain as biomechanics is to the body.

Our thoughts are not actually happening but they do stimulate a chemical reaction as real as the actual experience. We are merely reliving an experience in our head. We are not our thoughts. When we learn how to consciously shift a bad-feeling thought to a better-feeling thought, we can better control our emotions. So if you are thinking negative thoughts often, those are the thoughts that will pop up most often in the autopilot (unconscious). The same applies for positive thought.

> *"Think of your brain as the soil and your thoughts as the*
> *seeds. Which would you plant, flowers or weeds?"*
> ~ *Unknown*

This is why it is important to consciously think positive thoughts, think optimistically, be hopeful, and be grateful. The way to do this is to consciously direct your thoughts in the direction of your desire. For example, let's say you're having anxiety about a social event that you have to attend that evening. If you start to think of the best outcome, you can imagine the good food, drinks, music, and great conversations that you could have. Shifting the automatic stressful thoughts to thoughts of the best-case scenario could begin to bring down your anxiety level and even allow you to look forward to the event. In this case, the desire was the best possible outcome.

> *"We cannot always control what goes on outside, but we can control what goes on inside. It's that simple."*
> *~ Unknown*

We have the choice to think positive or to think negative. When something negative or stressful happens to us, we have the choice to stay stuck in the problem or start thinking of the solution. One thought of a solution will lead to another, and on and on. However, we must influence it. Remember, the MonkeyBrain has an addiction to the worst-case scenario. We have to choose our thoughts of the best-case scenario. We now know that our thoughts have a much more powerful effect on brain chemistry, emotions, and behavior. This effect on chemistry governs the way we feel. The way that we feel plays a huge role on how we think, speak, and act. Therefore, negative thinking has negative effects on our health and behavior, and positive thinking has positive effects on our health and behavior.[48] Think about the last event in your life that you considered awful or bad. You probably dealt with it pretty well.

> *"If we examine our thoughts, we shall find them always occupied with the past and the future. We must choose the thoughts of the present."*
> *~ Blaise Pascal*

---

[48] Martin, What is Positive Psychology, psychologyabout.com.

But then you continue to think about what happened and continued to create stress on the brain and the body. We cannot change the circumstances or events that happen, but we can change the way we continue to think and feel about the situation. If we look deeper, that awareness will often allow us to realize that the awful or bad circumstance in life, such as the end of a relationship or the loss of a job, usually turn out to be a blessing in disguise.

However, we also stress out about waiting in lines, relationship and work issues, traffic, financial insecurities, and many other things in life that can trigger a cascade of negative thoughts. All of these negative thoughts affect our health and our emotions. If you feel it necessary, allow yourself to feel sad, angry, or any other negative feeling; just don't allow yourself to wallow in the mud for very long. Self-pity, if not reined in, will overcome your entire body and will manifest into more pain and suffering.

It is understood that we have more permanent losses, such as the loss of a loved one or even internalizing someone else's pain. But we should also allow for the process to end when we have gone through it. In these cases, we must find acceptance in the situation, as we cannot change those circumstances. But we can only change the way that we think and feel about it.

As mentioned in Part I, emotional memory attached to pain or fear can be recalled without your consent. It is the memory that pops in and out of our thoughts at any time. As a matter of fact, we have very little control of when those thoughts pop in and out. This is actually an incredible design to help us avoid reliving painful or fearful experiences again. For instance, once we burn ourselves on something, say a hot fire, it is stored long-term, or for life, so we don't do it again. Most of us will avoid a fire because of the fear of pain. This is an example of legitimate pain and fear, and will prevent us from bodily injury or even death.

However, emotional memory (thoughts of a negative situation), such as the loss of a loved one, a divorce, or a tragic accident, can be relived over and over, which will eventually cause imbalance and create physical and mental illness. We can continue to relive emotional pain and fear over and over again in our thoughts. We continue to burn ourselves with emotional pain hundreds if not thousands of times. This may sound crazy to you, and that is because it is crazy. The definition of insanity is not just a deranged state of mind; it is doing the same thing over and over and expecting a different outcome. This includes thinking stressful or negative thoughts over and over and expecting to feel better. It will not happen!

Most things in life are not just black or white. But chemically speaking, the chemicals that are triggered by positive or negative thoughts, are indeed black or white. The thought either triggers good-feeling chemicals are bad-feeling chemicals. We cannot be positive and negative at the same time. We cannot be conscious and unconscious at the same time, and we cannot laugh and cry at the same time. We are never happy and sad at the same time. We cannot love and hate at the same time. It is not possible. However, we do have degrees of these emotions, which can range from enthusiasm, enjoyment, and satisfaction, to boredom, anger, fear, and grief. These emotions are either positive or negative. My experience tells me most of us have more negative thoughts than positive thoughts, and most of us have more fearful thoughts of disease than we do good thoughts of health. The goal is to have more positive thoughts than negative ones. Once you become aware of your thinking, you can then choose to reframe to a better thought. For example, the stories in Chapter I are good examples of how to reframe stress or negative thought patterns.

> *"Don't wait until you feel positive to move*
> *forward. Act your way into feeling good."*
> *~ John Maxwell*

The bottom line is this: Negative thinking is a habit that can be changed. The way to do this is to reframe every negative thought that you recognize and shift it to a better thought. Use the shifting process and keep shifting in the positive direction until you feel better. If the negative thoughts arise again, focus on whatever task or thing you are doing and stay out of your head. Consciously focus on your daily activities. Be aware when doing all of them, big or small. Remember, when we are completely aware of the moment that we are in, observing the experience, the MonkeyBrain is temporarily caged. I will end it here with a quote from one of the greatest minds of all time and the founder of quantum mechanics, Albert Einstein. This quote says it all!

> *"The manner of thinking that created the problem*
> *cannot be the means by which to solve it."*
> *~ Albert Einstein*

Congratulations! Now that you better understand how the human system works, you are ready to begin the twenty-one-day challenge. The twenty-one-day journal provided in the next section is designed to help you implement your goals and plan of action. Document all of your activity for each discipline, as well as other areas designed to help you improve emotional stability. This can help you learn what stress-reducing techniques work best for you. Once you have completed the twenty-one-day challenge, I recommend that you continue to journal and keep doing all of the work that made you better. Remember, this is not just about being well; this is about *being better*. Good luck with your continued growth and development, and keep in mind, the reward only follows when we do the work. There is no magic pill. It takes committed action over time and continued maintenance in all areas.

## Filling in the Missing Pieces

The bottom line is, whether we have a creator or not, we are co-creating our lives now. We are responsible for our thoughts, our words, and our actions. A balanced life is dependent on our mental, physical, and spiritual health. *MonkeyBrain* shared many ways to help create that balance. I hope the information helped you understand the entire human system and how each part works independently and with one another. The tools, techniques, and exercises that have been provided all improve, correct, or strengthen that specific discipline.

The fusion protocol is designed to change the chemical makeup of the brain while improving the physical body and brain function. The specific structure of the fusion addresses the entire human system. It is designed to improve brain function, challenge and strengthen the physical body, and develop spiritual awareness. Below is a list of activities or behaviors that improve each area. Use one or several activities for each area. Begin with short-term, small goals. As you reach your small goals, reset the next goals, and on and on. Should you not reach your goals, give yourself credit for what you have accomplished and keep striving for the same goal until you achieve it. You don't have to be better than anyone except for the person you were the day before. This isn't a competition; it's only a challenge for you.

> *"You are the one who can stretch your own horizon."*
> ~ *Edgar F. Magnin*

Choose one or more activities for each area. Improvement and change can be difficult at times. The twenty-one-day challenge is designed to help you stay focused and motivated. It provides structure. The journal allows you to see improvement, progression, and end results. This allows you to make changes at any time to improve or reset your program. Life in general may create challenges to your schedule, commitment, and goals. Modify your goals when needed.

## Brain Work

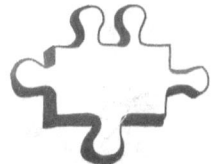

Learn new information
Learn a new skill
Do crossword or jigsaw puzzles
Do computer brain training
Do memory work
Find solutions to problems
Read
Write
Focus
Concentrate
Practice physical balance work

## Body Work

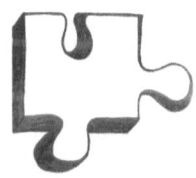

Proper movement
Balanced nutrition
Sufficient rest and sleep
Sufficient water

## Spirit/Mind Work

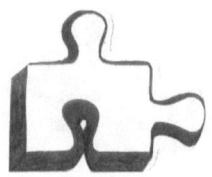

Love
Meditation
Prayer
Yoga/tai chi
Compassion
Forgiveness
Empathy
Trust
Acceptance
Maternal and Pair Bonding
Acts of service
Gratitude
Positive thinking
Creative work
Touch
(The following also activate the PNS, similar to other spiritual practices mentioned)
Music, scents, rhythmic dance, chants, mantras
Pets, flowers, sunsets, raw nature
Orgasm

The following is an example of a completed journal. Included are twenty-one blank days for you to begin journaling your participation. The twenty-one-day challenge can help you improve in whatever area needs work. Good luck, and just take it one day at a time.

*"Inch by inch, life is a cinch. Yard by yard, life is hard"*
*~ Unknown*

## The Joyefit Fusion™
## 21 Day Challenge

| Name: *John Doe* | Date: 5-1-14 | Weight: 175 |
|---|---|---|

### BRAIN TRAINING (list activity)

| | |
|---|---|
| 1. Read one chapter of new book | Duration: 20 minutes |
| 2. Cooking a new recipe for dinner tonight | Duration: 20 minutes |
| 3. *Spent 20 minutes playing video* | Duration: |

### Emotional Check List: (*GOOD – FAIR – POOR*)

| Energy: **Good** | Attitude: **Good** | Mood: **Good** |
|---|---|---|
| Motivation/Drive: **Good** | Stress Level: **fair** | Sleep: **Good** |

(List stressful events and ways that you were able to reduce the stress)

| Stress coping: |
|---|
| 1. My car broke down but I was able to drop it off so it can be repaired. |
| 2. Traffic was bad this evening so I played some chill music. I actually enjoyed my drive home from work today |

### BODY
### Physical Activity (*list specific activity*)

| Strength Training: **Total body w/ free weights** | Duration: **25 minutes** |
|---|---|
| Cardiovascular: **Cycling** | Duration: **20 minutes** |
| Flexibility: **Yoga** | Duration: **20 minutes** |
| Core Conditioning: **Included with Yoga** | Duration: **incl** |
| Other: | Duration: |

### Food Log:

| |
|---|
| Breakfast: **flax seed pita, 2 tbsp. peanut butter, 1 tbsp. honey, milk, coffee, water** |
| Snack: **20 gram protein, low carb shake** |
| Lunch: **4 oz deli chicken, whole grain pita, lettuce, tomatoes, onions, mustard. With mixed green salad and 1 cup of bean soup** |
| Snack: **1 apple and a hand full of peanuts** |
| Dinner: **8 oz. seared tuna, serving of green beans, mushrooms, onions. Decaf iced tea** |
| Water Intake: (oz.) **32** |

**SPIRIT**

**Spiritual development** (list specific activity)

| |
|---|
| Meditation: *spent quiet time for 5 minutes (fusion)* |
| Acts of service: *Spent time caring for Mom* |
| Forgiveness: |
| Acceptance: |
| Patience: *all day at work* |
| Compassion: *Gave a homeless man a few bucks for some food* |
| Prayer: *5 minutes quiet time before bed* |
| Touch: *hugged everyone that I worked with today and did 2 massages* |

| |
|---|
| Creative Projects: |
| |
| *Painting my bedroom and changing the look* |
| *Practicing drawing – sketching (or any other creative project)* |

**Gratitude Log:**

| |
|---|
| 1. *I'm so grateful for a great night sleep, because I feel great today.* |
| 2. *I'm very thankful for the new clients that I received today because it motivates me to work harder.* |
| 3. *I am so grateful for my motivation to work out today because I feel so much better when I exercise.* |
| 4. and so on |

**Daily Goals/Intentions** (*scratch off each one once accomplished*)

| |
|---|
| 1. *Eat healthy balanced meals and follow the fusion workout.* |
| 2. *Finish my work project and sign up a new client.* |
| 3. *Wash/dry and fold laundry* |

**Check the following for YES:**

| Vitamins: | Amino Acids: | Minerals: | Herbs: |
|---|---|---|---|
| | | | |

**NOTES:**

| |
|---|
| |
| |
| |

## The Joyefit Fusion™
## 21 Day Challenge

| Name: | Date: | Weight: |
|---|---|---|
| | | |

**BRAIN TRAINING (list activity)**

| 1. | Duration: |
|---|---|
| 2. | Duration: |
| 3. | Duration: |

**Emotional Check List:** (*GOOD – FAIR – POOR*)

| Energy: | Attitude: | Mood: |
|---|---|---|
| Motivation/Drive: | Stress Level: | Sleep: |

(List stressful events and ways that you were able to reduce the stress)

| Stress coping: |
|---|
| 1. |
| 2. |

**BODY**
**Physical Activity** (*list specific activity*)

| Strength Training: | Duration: |
|---|---|
| Cardiovascular: | Duration: |
| Flexibility: | Duration: |
| Core Conditioning: | Duration: |
| Other: | Duration: |

**Food Log:**

| Breakfast: |
|---|
| |

190

| |
|---|
| Snack: |
| Lunch: |
| Snack: |
| Dinner: |
| Water Intake: (oz.) |

**SPIRIT**
**Spiritual development** (list specific activity)

| |
|---|
| Meditation: |
| Acts of service: |
| Forgiveness: |
| Acceptance: |
| Patience: |
| Compassion: |
| Prayer: |
| Touch: |

| |
|---|
| Creative Projects: |
| |

**Gratitude Log:**

| |
|---|
| 1. |
| 2. |
| 3. |
| 4. |
| 5. |

**Daily Goals/Intentions** (*scratch off each one once accomplished*)

| |
|---|
| 1. |
| 2. |
| 3. |

**Check the following for YES:**

| Vitamins: ☐ | Amino Acids: ☐ | Minerals: ☐ | Herbs: ☐ |
|---|---|---|---|

**NOTES:**

| |
|---|
| |
| ADDL: |

## The Joyefit Fusion™
### Day 2

| Name: | Date: | Weight: |
|-------|-------|---------|
|       |       |         |

**BRAIN TRAINING (list activity)**

| 1. | Duration: |
|----|-----------|
| 2. | Duration: |
| 3. | Duration: |

**Emotional Check List:** (*GOOD – FAIR – POOR*)

| Energy: | Attitude: | Mood: |
|---------|-----------|-------|
| Motivation/Drive: | Stress Level: | Sleep: |

(List stressful events and ways that you were able to reduce the stress)

| Stress coping: |
|----------------|
| 1. |
| 2. |

**BODY**
**Physical Activity** (*list specific activity*)

| Strength Training: | Duration: |
|--------------------|-----------|
| Cardiovascular: | Duration: |
| Flexibility: | Duration: |
| Core Conditioning: | Duration: |
| Other: | Duration: |

**Food Log:**

| Breakfast: |
|------------|

| |
|---|
| Snack: |
| Lunch: |
| Snack: |
| Dinner: |
| Water Intake: (oz.) |

**SPIRIT**
**Spiritual development** (list specific activity)

| |
|---|
| Meditation: |
| Acts of service: |
| Forgiveness: |
| Acceptance: |
| Patience: |
| Compassion: |
| Prayer: |
| Touch: |

| |
|---|
| Creative Projects: |

**Gratitude Log:**

| | |
|---|---|
| 1. | |
| 2. | |
| 3. | |
| 4. | |
| 5. | |

**Daily Goals/Intentions** (*scratch off each one once accomplished*)

| | |
|---|---|
| 1. | |
| 2. | |
| 3. | |

**Check the following for YES:**

| Vitamins: ☐ | Amino Acids: ☐ | Minerals: ☐ | Herbs: ☐ |
|---|---|---|---|

**NOTES:**

ADDL:

# The Joyefit Fusion™
## Day 3

| Name: | Date: | Weight: |
|---|---|---|
| | | |

**BRAIN TRAINING (list activity)**

| 1. | Duration: |
|---|---|
| 2. | Duration: |
| 3. | Duration: |

**Emotional Check List:** (*GOOD – FAIR – POOR*)

| Energy: | Attitude: | Mood: |
|---|---|---|
| Motivation/Drive: | Stress Level: | Sleep: |

(List stressful events and ways that you were able to reduce the stress)

| Stress coping:<br>1.<br>2. |
|---|

**BODY**

**Physical Activity** (*list specific activity*)

| Strength Training: | Duration: |
|---|---|
| Cardiovascular: | Duration: |
| Flexibility: | Duration: |
| Core Conditioning: | Duration: |
| Other: | Duration: |

**Food Log:**

| Breakfast: |
|---|

| |
|---|
| Snack: |
| Lunch: |
| Snack: |
| Dinner: |
| Water Intake: (oz.) |

**SPIRIT**
**Spiritual development** (list specific activity)

| |
|---|
| Meditation: |
| Acts of service: |
| Forgiveness: |
| Acceptance: |
| Patience: |
| Compassion: |
| Prayer: |
| Touch: |

| |
|---|
| Creative Projects: |

**Gratitude Log:**

| |
|---|
| 1. |
| 2. |
| 3. |
| 4. |
| 5. |

**Daily Goals/Intentions** (*scratch off each one once accomplished*)

| |
|---|
| 1. |
| 2. |
| 3. |

**Check the following for YES:**

| Vitamins: ☐ | Amino Acids: ☐ | Minerals: ☐ | Herbs: ☐ |
|---|---|---|---|

**NOTES:**

| |
|---|
| |
| |
| |
| |
| |
| |
| ADDL: |

# The Joyefit Fusion™
## Day 4

| Name: | Date: | Weight: |
|---|---|---|
|  |  |  |

**BRAIN TRAINING (list activity)**

| 1. | Duration: |
|---|---|
| 2. | Duration: |
| 3. | Duration: |

**Emotional Check List:** (*GOOD – FAIR – POOR*)

| Energy: | Attitude: | Mood: |
|---|---|---|
| Motivation/Drive: | Stress Level: | Sleep: |

(List stressful events and ways that you were able to reduce the stress)

| Stress coping: |
|---|
| 1. |
| 2. |

**BODY**

**Physical Activity** (*list specific activity*)

| Strength Training: | Duration: |
|---|---|
| Cardiovascular: | Duration: |
| Flexibility: | Duration: |
| Core Conditioning: | Duration: |
| Other: | Duration: |

**Food Log:**

| Breakfast: |
|---|

| Snack: |
| Lunch: |
| Snack: |
| Dinner: |
| Water Intake: (oz.) |

**SPIRIT**
**Spiritual development** (list specific activity)

| Meditation: |
| Acts of service: |
| Forgiveness: |
| Acceptance: |
| Patience: |
| Compassion: |
| Prayer: |
| Touch: |

| Creative Projects: |

**Gratitude Log:**

| | |
|---|---|
| 1. | |
| 2. | |
| 3. | |
| 4. | |
| 5. | |

**Daily Goals/Intentions** (*scratch off each one once accomplished*)

| | |
|---|---|
| 1. | |
| 2. | |
| 3. | |

**Check the following for YES:**

| Vitamins: ☐ | Amino Acids: ☐ | Minerals: ☐ | Herbs: ☐ |
|---|---|---|---|

**NOTES:**

ADDL:

# The Joyefit Fusion™
## Day 5

| Name: | Date: | Weight: |
|---|---|---|
|  |  |  |

**BRAIN TRAINING (list activity)**

| 1. | Duration: |
|---|---|
| 2. | Duration: |
| 3. | Duration: |

**Emotional Check List:** (*GOOD – FAIR – POOR*)

| Energy: | Attitude: | Mood: |
|---|---|---|
| Motivation/Drive: | Stress Level: | Sleep: |

(List stressful events and ways that you were able to reduce the stress)

| Stress coping:<br>1.<br>2. |
|---|

**BODY**
**Physical Activity** (*list specific activity*)

| Strength Training: | Duration: |
|---|---|
| Cardiovascular: | Duration: |
| Flexibility: | Duration: |
| Core Conditioning: | Duration: |
| Other: | Duration: |

**Food Log:**

| Breakfast: |
|---|

| |
|---|
| Snack: |
| Lunch: |
| Snack: |
| Dinner: |
| Water Intake: (oz.) |

**SPIRIT**
**Spiritual development** (list specific activity)

| |
|---|
| Meditation: |
| Acts of service: |
| Forgiveness: |
| Acceptance: |
| Patience: |
| Compassion: |
| Prayer: |
| Touch: |

| |
|---|
| Creative Projects: |

**Gratitude Log:**

| |
|---|
| 1. |
| 2. |
| 3. |
| 4. |
| 5. |

**Daily Goals/Intentions** (*scratch off each one once accomplished*)

| |
|---|
| 1. |
| 2. |
| 3. |

**Check the following for YES:**

| Vitamins: ☐ | Amino Acids: ☐ | Minerals: ☐ | Herbs: ☐ |
|---|---|---|---|

**NOTES:**

| |
|---|
| |
| |
| |
| |
| |
| |
| |
| ADDL: |

## The Joyefit Fusion™
### Day 6

| Name: | Date: | Weight: |
|-------|-------|---------|
|       |       |         |

**BRAIN TRAINING (list activity)**

| 1. | Duration: |
|----|-----------|
| 2. | Duration: |
| 3. | Duration: |

**Emotional Check List:** (*GOOD – FAIR – POOR*)

| Energy: | Attitude: | Mood: |
|---------|-----------|-------|
| Motivation/Drive: | Stress Level: | Sleep: |

(List stressful events and ways that you were able to reduce the stress)

| Stress coping:<br>1.<br>2. |
|---|

**BODY**

**Physical Activity** (*list specific activity*)

| Strength Training: | Duration: |
|--------------------|-----------|
| Cardiovascular: | Duration: |
| Flexibility: | Duration: |
| Core Conditioning: | Duration: |
| Other: | Duration: |

**Food Log:**

| Breakfast: |
|---|

| |
|---|
| Snack: |
| Lunch: |
| Snack: |
| Dinner: |
| Water Intake: (oz.) |

**SPIRIT**

**Spiritual development** (list specific activity)

| |
|---|
| Meditation: |
| Acts of service: |
| Forgiveness: |
| Acceptance: |
| Patience: |
| Compassion: |
| Prayer: |
| Touch: |

| |
|---|
| Creative Projects: |

**Gratitude Log:**

| |
|---|
| 1. |
| 2. |
| 3. |
| 4. |
| 5. |

**Daily Goals/Intentions** (*scratch off each one once accomplished*)

| |
|---|
| 1. |
| 2. |
| 3. |

**Check the following for YES:**

| Vitamins: ☐ | Amino Acids: ☐ | Minerals: ☐ | Herbs: ☐ |
|---|---|---|---|

**NOTES:**

| |
|---|
| |
| |
| |
| |
| |
| |
| ADDL: |

## The Joyefit Fusion™
### Day 7

| Name: | Date: | Weight: |
|---|---|---|
| | | |

**BRAIN TRAINING (list activity)**

| | |
|---|---|
| 1. | Duration: |
| 2. | Duration: |
| 3. | Duration: |

**Emotional Check List:** (*GOOD – FAIR – POOR*)

| Energy: | Attitude: | Mood: |
|---|---|---|
| Motivation/Drive: | Stress Level: | Sleep: |

(List stressful events and ways that you were able to reduce the stress)

| |
|---|
| Stress coping:<br>1.<br>2. |

**BODY**

**Physical Activity** (*list specific activity*)

| | |
|---|---|
| Strength Training: | Duration: |
| Cardiovascular: | Duration: |
| Flexibility: | Duration: |
| Core Conditioning: | Duration: |
| Other: | Duration: |

**Food Log:**

| |
|---|
| Breakfast: |

| |
|---|
| Snack: |
| Lunch: |
| Snack: |
| Dinner: |
| Water Intake: (oz.) |

**SPIRIT**
**Spiritual development** (list specific activity)

| |
|---|
| Meditation: |
| Acts of service: |
| Forgiveness: |
| Acceptance: |
| Patience: |
| Compassion: |
| Prayer: |
| Touch: |

| |
|---|
| Creative Projects: |

**Gratitude Log:**

| |
|---|
| 1. |
| 2. |
| 3. |
| 4. |
| 5. |

**Daily Goals/Intentions** (*scratch off each one once accomplished*)

| |
|---|
| 1. |
| 2. |
| 3. |

**Check the following for YES:**

| Vitamins: ☐ | Amino Acids: ☐ | Minerals: ☐ | Herbs: ☐ |
|---|---|---|---|

**NOTES:**

| |
|---|
| |
| |
| |
| |
| |
| |
| ADDL: |

## The Joyefit Fusion™
## Day 8

| Name: | Date: | Weight: |
|---|---|---|
| | | |

**BRAIN TRAINING (list activity)**

| | |
|---|---|
| 1. | Duration: |
| 2. | Duration: |
| 3. | Duration: |

**Emotional Check List:** (*GOOD – FAIR – POOR*)

| | | |
|---|---|---|
| Energy: | Attitude: | Mood: |
| Motivation/Drive: | Stress Level: | Sleep: |

(List stressful events and ways that you were able to reduce the stress)

| |
|---|
| Stress coping: |
| 1. |
| 2. |

**BODY**

**Physical Activity** (*list specific activity*)

| | |
|---|---|
| Strength Training: | Duration: |
| Cardiovascular: | Duration: |
| Flexibility: | Duration: |
| Core Conditioning: | Duration: |
| Other: | Duration: |

**Food Log:**

| |
|---|
| Breakfast: |

| |
|---|
| Snack: |
| Lunch: |
| Snack: |
| Dinner: |
| Water Intake: (oz.) |

**SPIRIT**

**Spiritual development** (list specific activity)

| |
|---|
| Meditation: |
| Acts of service: |
| Forgiveness: |
| Acceptance: |
| Patience: |
| Compassion: |
| Prayer: |
| Touch: |

| |
|---|
| Creative Projects: |

**Gratitude Log:**

| |
|---|
| 1. |
| 2. |
| 3. |
| 4. |
| 5. |

**Daily Goals/Intentions** (*scratch off each one once accomplished*)

| |
|---|
| 1. |
| 2. |
| 3. |

**Check the following for YES:**

| Vitamins: ☐ | Amino Acids: ☐ | Minerals: ☐ | Herbs: ☐ |
|---|---|---|---|

**NOTES:**

ADDL:

## The Joyefit Fusion™
### Day 9

| Name: | Date: | Weight: |
|---|---|---|
|  |  |  |

**BRAIN TRAINING (list activity)**

| 1. | Duration: |
|---|---|
| 2. | Duration: |
| 3. | Duration: |

**Emotional Check List:** (*GOOD – FAIR – POOR*)

| Energy: | Attitude: | Mood: |
|---|---|---|
| Motivation/Drive: | Stress Level: | Sleep: |

(List stressful events and ways that you were able to reduce the stress)

| Stress coping:<br>1.<br>2. |
|---|

**BODY**

**Physical Activity** (*list specific activity*)

| Strength Training: | Duration: |
|---|---|
| Cardiovascular: | Duration: |
| Flexibility: | Duration: |
| Core Conditioning: | Duration: |
| Other: | Duration: |

**Food Log:**

| Breakfast: |
|---|

| |
|---|
| Snack: |
| Lunch: |
| Snack: |
| Dinner: |
| Water Intake: (oz.) |

**SPIRIT**
**Spiritual development** (list specific activity)

| |
|---|
| Meditation: |
| Acts of service: |
| Forgiveness: |
| Acceptance: |
| Patience: |
| Compassion: |
| Prayer: |
| Touch: |

| |
|---|
| Creative Projects: |

**Gratitude Log:**

| 1. |
|---|
| 2. |
| 3. |
| 4. |
| 5. |

**Daily Goals/Intentions** (*scratch off each one once accomplished*)

| 1. |
|---|
| 2. |
| 3. |

**Check the following for YES:**

| Vitamins: ☐ | Amino Acids: ☐ | Minerals: ☐ | Herbs: ☐ |
|---|---|---|---|

**NOTES:**

|  |
|---|
|  |

ADDL:

## The Joyefit Fusion™
## Day 10

| Name: | Date: | Weight: |
|---|---|---|
| | | |

**BRAIN TRAINING (list activity)**

| 1. | Duration: |
|---|---|
| 2. | Duration: |
| 3. | Duration: |

**Emotional Check List:** (*GOOD – FAIR – POOR*)

| Energy: | Attitude: | Mood: |
|---|---|---|
| Motivation/Drive: | Stress Level: | Sleep: |

(List stressful events and ways that you were able to reduce the stress)

| Stress coping: |
|---|
| 1. |
| 2. |

**BODY**

**Physical Activity** (*list specific activity*)

| Strength Training: | Duration: |
|---|---|
| Cardiovascular: | Duration: |
| Flexibility: | Duration: |
| Core Conditioning: | Duration: |
| Other: | Duration: |

**Food Log:**

| Breakfast: |
|---|

| |
|---|
| Snack: |
| Lunch: |
| Snack: |
| Dinner: |
| Water Intake: (oz.) |

**SPIRIT**
**Spiritual development** (list specific activity)

| |
|---|
| Meditation: |
| Acts of service: |
| Forgiveness: |
| Acceptance: |
| Patience: |
| Compassion: |
| Prayer: |
| Touch: |

| |
|---|
| Creative Projects: |

**Gratitude Log:**

| 1. |
|---|
| 2. |
| 3. |
| 4. |
| 5. |

**Daily Goals/Intentions** *(scratch off each one once accomplished)*

| 1. |
|---|
| 2. |
| 3. |

**Check the following for YES:**

| Vitamins: ☐ | Amino Acids: ☐ | Minerals: ☐ | Herbs: ☐ |
|---|---|---|---|

**NOTES:**

ADDL:

## The Joyefit Fusion™
## Day 11

| Name: | Date: | Weight: |
|---|---|---|
|  |  |  |

**BRAIN TRAINING (list activity)**

| | |
|---|---|
| 1. | Duration: |
| 2. | Duration: |
| 3. | Duration: |

**Emotional Check List:** (*GOOD – FAIR – POOR*)

| Energy: | Attitude: | Mood: |
|---|---|---|
| Motivation/Drive: | Stress Level: | Sleep: |

(List stressful events and ways that you were able to reduce the stress)

| |
|---|
| Stress coping: |
| 1. |
| 2. |

**BODY**

**Physical Activity** (*list specific activity*)

| | |
|---|---|
| Strength Training: | Duration: |
| Cardiovascular: | Duration: |
| Flexibility: | Duration: |
| Core Conditioning: | Duration: |
| Other: | Duration: |

**Food Log:**

| |
|---|
| Breakfast: |

| |
|---|
| Snack: |
| Lunch: |
| Snack: |
| Dinner: |
| Water Intake: (oz.) |

**SPIRIT**
**Spiritual development** (list specific activity)

| |
|---|
| Meditation: |
| Acts of service: |
| Forgiveness: |
| Acceptance: |
| Patience: |
| Compassion: |
| Prayer: |
| Touch: |

| |
|---|
| Creative Projects: |
| |

**Gratitude Log:**

| | |
|---|---|
| 1. | |
| 2. | |
| 3. | |
| 4. | |
| 5. | |

**Daily Goals/Intentions** (*scratch off each one once accomplished*)

| | |
|---|---|
| 1. | |
| 2. | |
| 3. | |

**Check the following for YES:**

| Vitamins: ☐ | Amino Acids: ☐ | Minerals: ☐ | Herbs: ☐ |
|---|---|---|---|

**NOTES:**

ADDL:

# The Joyefit Fusion™
## Day 12

| Name: | Date: | Weight: |
|-------|-------|---------|
|       |       |         |

**BRAIN TRAINING (list activity)**

| 1. | Duration: |
|----|-----------|
| 2. | Duration: |
| 3. | Duration: |

**Emotional Check List:** (*GOOD – FAIR – POOR*)

| Energy: | Attitude: | Mood: |
|---------|-----------|-------|
| Motivation/Drive: | Stress Level: | Sleep: |

(List stressful events and ways that you were able to reduce the stress)

| Stress coping:<br>1.<br>2. |
|----|

**BODY**
**Physical Activity** (*list specific activity*)

| Strength Training: | Duration: |
|--------------------|-----------|
| Cardiovascular: | Duration: |
| Flexibility: | Duration: |
| Core Conditioning: | Duration: |
| Other: | Duration: |

**Food Log:**

| Breakfast: |
|------------|

| |
|---|
| Snack: |
| Lunch: |
| Snack: |
| Dinner: |
| Water Intake: (oz.) |

**SPIRIT**
**Spiritual development** (list specific activity)

| |
|---|
| Meditation: |
| Acts of service: |
| Forgiveness: |
| Acceptance: |
| Patience: |
| Compassion: |
| Prayer: |
| Touch: |

| |
|---|
| Creative Projects: |

**Gratitude Log:**

| 1. |
|---|
| 2. |
| 3. |
| 4. |
| 5. |

**Daily Goals/Intentions** (*scratch off each one once accomplished*)

| 1. |
|---|
| 2. |
| 3. |

**Check the following for YES:**

| Vitamins: ☐ | Amino Acids: ☐ | Minerals: ☐ | Herbs: ☐ |
|---|---|---|---|

**NOTES:**

ADDL:

## The Joyefit Fusion™
## Day 13

| Name: | Date: | Weight: |
|---|---|---|
|  |  |  |

**BRAIN TRAINING (list activity)**

| 1. | Duration: |
|---|---|
| 2. | Duration: |
| 3. | Duration: |

**Emotional Check List:** (*GOOD – FAIR – POOR*)

| Energy: | Attitude: | Mood: |
|---|---|---|
| Motivation/Drive: | Stress Level: | Sleep: |

(List stressful events and ways that you were able to reduce the stress)

| Stress coping: |
|---|
| 1. |
| 2. |

**BODY**
**Physical Activity** (*list specific activity*)

| Strength Training: | Duration: |
|---|---|
| Cardiovascular: | Duration: |
| Flexibility: | Duration: |
| Core Conditioning: | Duration: |
| Other: | Duration: |

**Food Log:**

| Breakfast: |
|---|

| |
|---|
| Snack: |
| Lunch: |
| Snack: |
| Dinner: |
| Water Intake: (oz.) |

**SPIRIT**
**Spiritual development** (list specific activity)

| |
|---|
| Meditation: |
| Acts of service: |
| Forgiveness: |
| Acceptance: |
| Patience: |
| Compassion: |
| Prayer: |
| Touch: |

| |
|---|
| Creative Projects: |

**Gratitude Log:**

| | |
|---|---|
| 1. | |
| 2. | |
| 3. | |
| 4. | |
| 5. | |

**Daily Goals/Intentions** (*scratch off each one once accomplished*)

| | |
|---|---|
| 1. | |
| 2. | |
| 3. | |

**Check the following for YES:**

| Vitamins: ☐ | Amino Acids: ☐ | Minerals: ☐ | Herbs: ☐ |
|---|---|---|---|

**NOTES:**

| |
|---|
| |
| |
| |
| |
| |
| |
| |
| ADDL: |
| |

## The Joyefit Fusion™
## Day 14

| Name: | Date: | Weight: |
|---|---|---|
| | | |

**BRAIN TRAINING (list activity)**

| | |
|---|---|
| 1. | Duration: |
| 2. | Duration: |
| 3. | Duration: |

**Emotional Check List:** (*GOOD – FAIR – POOR*)

| Energy: | Attitude: | Mood: |
|---|---|---|
| Motivation/Drive: | Stress Level: | Sleep: |

(List stressful events and ways that you were able to reduce the stress)

| |
|---|
| Stress coping: |
| 1. |
| 2. |

**BODY**

**Physical Activity** (*list specific activity*)

| | |
|---|---|
| Strength Training: | Duration: |
| Cardiovascular: | Duration: |
| Flexibility: | Duration: |
| Core Conditioning: | Duration: |
| Other: | Duration: |

**Food Log:**

| |
|---|
| Breakfast: |

| |
|---|
| Snack: |
| Lunch: |
| Snack: |
| Dinner: |
| Water Intake: (oz.) |

**SPIRIT**

**Spiritual development** (list specific activity)

| |
|---|
| Meditation: |
| |
| Acts of service: |
| |
| Forgiveness: |
| |
| Acceptance: |
| |
| Patience: |
| |
| Compassion: |
| |
| Prayer: |
| |
| Touch: |
| |

| |
|---|
| Creative Projects: |
| |
| |

**Gratitude Log:**

| |
|---|
| 1. |
| 2. |
| 3. |
| 4. |
| 5. |

**Daily Goals/Intentions** *(scratch off each one once accomplished)*

| |
|---|
| 1. |
| 2. |
| 3. |

**Check the following for YES:**

| Vitamins: ☐ | Amino Acids: ☐ | Minerals: ☐ | Herbs: ☐ |
|---|---|---|---|

**NOTES:**

| |
|---|
| |
| |
| |
| |
| |
| |
| ADDL: |

## The Joyefit Fusion™
### Day 15

| Name: | Date: | Weight: |
|-------|-------|---------|
|       |       |         |

**BRAIN TRAINING (list activity)**

| 1. | Duration: |
|----|-----------|
| 2. | Duration: |
| 3. | Duration: |

**Emotional Check List:** (*GOOD – FAIR – POOR*)

| Energy: | Attitude: | Mood: |
|---------|-----------|-------|
| Motivation/Drive: | Stress Level: | Sleep: |

(List stressful events and ways that you were able to reduce the stress)

| Stress coping: |
|----------------|
| 1. |
| 2. |

**BODY**

**Physical Activity** (*list specific activity*)

| Strength Training: | Duration: |
|--------------------|-----------|
| Cardiovascular: | Duration: |
| Flexibility: | Duration: |
| Core Conditioning: | Duration: |
| Other: | Duration: |

**Food Log:**

| Breakfast: |
|------------|
|            |

| |
|---|
| Snack: |
| Lunch: |
| Snack: |
| Dinner: |
| Water Intake: (oz.) |

**SPIRIT**
**Spiritual development** (list specific activity)

| |
|---|
| Meditation: |
| Acts of service: |
| Forgiveness: |
| Acceptance: |
| Patience: |
| Compassion: |
| Prayer: |
| Touch: |

| |
|---|
| Creative Projects: |

**Gratitude Log:**

| |
|---|
| 1. |
| 2. |
| 3. |
| 4. |
| 5. |

**Daily Goals/Intentions** (*scratch off each one once accomplished*)

| |
|---|
| 1. |
| 2. |
| 3. |

**Check the following for YES:**

| Vitamins: ☐ | Amino Acids: ☐ | Minerals: ☐ | Herbs: ☐ |
|---|---|---|---|

**NOTES:**

ADDL:

## *The Joyefit Fusion™*
## *Day 16*

| Name: | Date: | Weight: |
|---|---|---|
| | | |

**BRAIN TRAINING (list activity)**

| | |
|---|---|
| 1. | Duration: |
| 2. | Duration: |
| 3. | Duration: |

**Emotional Check List:** (*GOOD – FAIR – POOR*)

| | | |
|---|---|---|
| Energy: | Attitude: | Mood: |
| Motivation/Drive: | Stress Level: | Sleep: |

(List stressful events and ways that you were able to reduce the stress)

| Stress coping: |
|---|
| 1. |
| 2. |

**BODY**

**Physical Activity** (*list specific activity*)

| | |
|---|---|
| Strength Training: | Duration: |
| Cardiovascular: | Duration: |
| Flexibility: | Duration: |
| Core Conditioning: | Duration: |
| Other: | Duration: |

**Food Log:**

| Breakfast: |
|---|

| |
|---|
| Snack: |
| Lunch: |
| Snack: |
| Dinner: |
| Water Intake: (oz.) |

**SPIRIT**
**Spiritual development** (list specific activity)

| |
|---|
| Meditation: |
| Acts of service: |
| Forgiveness: |
| Acceptance: |
| Patience: |
| Compassion: |
| Prayer: |
| Touch: |

| |
|---|
| Creative Projects: |
| |

**Gratitude Log:**

| |
|---|
| 1. |
| 2. |
| 3. |
| 4. |
| 5. |

**Daily Goals/Intentions** (*scratch off each one once accomplished*)

| |
|---|
| 1. |
| 2. |
| 3. |

**Check the following for YES:**

| | | | |
|---|---|---|---|
| Vitamins: ☐ | Amino Acids: ☐ | Minerals: ☐ | Herbs: ☐ |

**NOTES:**

| |
|---|
| |

ADDL:

| Name: | Date: | Weight: |
|---|---|---|
|  |  |  |

**BRAIN TRAINING (list activity)**

| 1. | Duration: |
|---|---|
| 2. | Duration: |
| 3. | Duration: |

**Emotional Check List:** (*GOOD – FAIR – POOR*)

| Energy: | Attitude: | Mood: |
|---|---|---|
| Motivation/Drive: | Stress Level: | Sleep: |

(List stressful events and ways that you were able to reduce the stress)

| Stress coping: |
|---|
| 1. |
| 2. |

**BODY**

**Physical Activity** (*list specific activity*)

| Strength Training: | Duration: |
|---|---|
| Cardiovascular: | Duration: |
| Flexibility: | Duration: |
| Core Conditioning: | Duration: |
| Other: | Duration: |

**Food Log:**

| Breakfast: |
|---|
|  |

| |
|---|
| Snack: |
| Lunch: |
| Snack: |
| Dinner: |
| Water Intake: (oz.) |

**SPIRIT**
**Spiritual development** (list specific activity)

| |
|---|
| Meditation: |
| Acts of service: |
| Forgiveness: |
| Acceptance: |
| Patience: |
| Compassion: |
| Prayer: |
| Touch: |

| |
|---|
| Creative Projects: |
| |

**Gratitude Log:**

| 1. |
|---|
| 2. |
| 3. |
| 4. |
| 5. |

**Daily Goals/Intentions** (*scratch off each one once accomplished*)

| 1. |
|---|
| 2. |
| 3. |

**Check the following for YES:**

| Vitamins: ☐ | Amino Acids: ☐ | Minerals: ☐ | Herbs: ☐ |
|---|---|---|---|

**NOTES:**

|  |
|---|
|  |
|  |
|  |
|  |
|  |
|  |
| ADDL: |

## The Joyefit Fusion™
## Day 18

| Name: | Date: | Weight: |
|---|---|---|
|  |  |  |

**BRAIN TRAINING (list activity)**

| 1. | Duration: |
|---|---|
| 2. | Duration: |
| 3. | Duration: |

**Emotional Check List:** (*GOOD – FAIR – POOR*)

| Energy: | Attitude: | Mood: |
|---|---|---|
| Motivation/Drive: | Stress Level: | Sleep: |

(List stressful events and ways that you were able to reduce the stress)

| Stress coping: |
|---|
| 1. |
| 2. |

**BODY**

**Physical Activity** (*list specific activity*)

| Strength Training: | Duration: |
|---|---|
| Cardiovascular: | Duration: |
| Flexibility: | Duration: |
| Core Conditioning: | Duration: |
| Other: | Duration: |

**Food Log:**

| Breakfast: |
|---|

| |
|---|
| Snack: |
| Lunch: |
| Snack: |
| Dinner: |
| Water Intake: (oz.) |

**SPIRIT**
**Spiritual development** (list specific activity)

| |
|---|
| Meditation: |
| Acts of service: |
| Forgiveness: |
| Acceptance: |
| Patience: |
| Compassion: |
| Prayer: |
| Touch: |

| |
|---|
| Creative Projects: |
| |

**Gratitude Log:**

| |
|---|
| 1. |
| 2. |
| 3. |
| 4. |
| 5. |

**Daily Goals/Intentions** (*scratch off each one once accomplished*)

| |
|---|
| 1. |
| 2. |
| 3. |

**Check the following for YES:**

| Vitamins: □ | Amino Acids: □ | Minerals: □ | Herbs: □ |
|---|---|---|---|

**NOTES:**

| |
|---|
| |
| |
| |
| |
| |
| |
| ADDL: |

## The Joyefit Fusion™
### Day 19

| Name: | Date: | Weight: |
|-------|-------|---------|
|       |       |         |

### BRAIN TRAINING (list activity)

| 1. | Duration: |
|----|-----------|
| 2. | Duration: |
| 3. | Duration: |

### Emotional Check List: (GOOD – FAIR – POOR)

| Energy: | Attitude: | Mood: |
|---------|-----------|-------|
| Motivation/Drive: | Stress Level: | Sleep: |

(List stressful events and ways that you were able to reduce the stress)

| Stress coping:<br>1.<br>2. |
|---|

### BODY
### Physical Activity (list specific activity)

| Strength Training: | Duration: |
|--------------------|-----------|
| Cardiovascular: | Duration: |
| Flexibility: | Duration: |
| Core Conditioning: | Duration: |
| Other: | Duration: |

### Food Log:

| Breakfast: |
|---|

| |
|---|
| Snack: |
| Lunch: |
| Snack: |
| Dinner: |
| Water Intake: (oz.) |

**SPIRIT**

**Spiritual development** (list specific activity)

| |
|---|
| Meditation: |
| |
| Acts of service: |
| |
| Forgiveness: |
| |
| Acceptance: |
| |
| Patience: |
| |
| Compassion: |
| |
| Prayer: |
| |
| Touch: |
| |

| |
|---|
| Creative Projects: |
| |
| |

**Gratitude Log:**

| | |
|---|---|
| 1. | |
| 2. | |
| 3. | |
| 4. | |
| 5. | |

**Daily Goals/Intentions** (*scratch off each one once accomplished*)

| | |
|---|---|
| 1. | |
| 2. | |
| 3. | |

**Check the following for YES:**

| Vitamins: ☐ | Amino Acids: ☐ | Minerals: ☐ | Herbs: ☐ |
|---|---|---|---|

**NOTES:**

ADDL:

## The Joyefit Fusion™
## Day 20

| Name: | Date: | Weight: |
|-------|-------|---------|
|       |       |         |

**BRAIN TRAINING (list activity)**

| 1. | Duration: |
|----|-----------|
| 2. | Duration: |
| 3. | Duration: |

**Emotional Check List:** (*GOOD – FAIR – POOR*)

| Energy: | Attitude: | Mood: |
|---------|-----------|-------|
| Motivation/Drive: | Stress Level: | Sleep: |

(List stressful events and ways that you were able to reduce the stress)

| Stress coping: |
|----------------|
| 1. |
| 2. |

**BODY**
**Physical Activity** (*list specific activity*)

| Strength Training: | Duration: |
|--------------------|-----------|
| Cardiovascular: | Duration: |
| Flexibility: | Duration: |
| Core Conditioning: | Duration: |
| Other: | Duration: |

**Food Log:**

| Breakfast: |
|------------|
|            |

| |
|---|
| Snack: |
| Lunch: |
| Snack: |
| Dinner: |
| Water Intake: (oz.) |

**SPIRIT**
**Spiritual development** (list specific activity)

| |
|---|
| Meditation: |
| |
| Acts of service: |
| |
| Forgiveness: |
| |
| Acceptance: |
| |
| Patience: |
| |
| Compassion: |
| |
| Prayer: |
| |
| Touch: |
| |

| |
|---|
| Creative Projects: |
| |
| |

**Gratitude Log:**

| |
|---|
| 1. |
| 2. |
| 3. |
| 4. |
| 5. |

**Daily Goals/Intentions** *(scratch off each one once accomplished)*

| |
|---|
| 1. |
| 2. |
| 3. |

**Check the following for YES:**

| Vitamins: ☐ | Amino Acids: ☐ | Minerals: ☐ | Herbs: ☐ |
|---|---|---|---|

**NOTES:**

| |
|---|
| |
| |
| |
| |
| |
| |
| |
| ADDL: |

# The Joyefit Fusion™
## Day 21

| Name: | Date: | Weight: |
|---|---|---|
| | | |

**BRAIN TRAINING (list activity)**

| | |
|---|---|
| 1. | Duration: |
| 2. | Duration: |
| 3. | Duration: |

**Emotional Check List:** (*GOOD – FAIR – POOR*)

| Energy: | Attitude: | Mood: |
|---|---|---|
| Motivation/Drive: | Stress Level: | Sleep: |

(List stressful events and ways that you were able to reduce the stress)

| |
|---|
| Stress coping: |
| 1. |
| 2. |

**BODY**

**Physical Activity** (*list specific activity*)

| | |
|---|---|
| Strength Training: | Duration: |
| Cardiovascular: | Duration: |
| Flexibility: | Duration: |
| Core Conditioning: | Duration: |
| Other: | Duration: |

**Food Log:**

| |
|---|
| Breakfast: |

| |
|---|
| Snack: |
| Lunch: |
| Snack: |
| Dinner: |
| Water Intake: (oz.) |

**SPIRIT**
**Spiritual development** (list specific activity)

| |
|---|
| Meditation: |
| Acts of service: |
| Forgiveness: |
| Acceptance: |
| Patience: |
| Compassion: |
| Prayer: |
| Touch: |

| |
|---|
| Creative Projects: |
| |

**Gratitude Log:**

| |
|---|
| 1. |
| 2. |
| 3. |
| 4. |
| 5. |

**Daily Goals/Intentions** (*scratch off each one once accomplished*)

| |
|---|
| 1. |
| 2. |
| 3. |

**Check the following for YES:**

| Vitamins: ☐ | Amino Acids: ☐ | Minerals: ☐ | Herbs: ☐ |
|---|---|---|---|

**NOTES:**

| |
|---|
| |
| |
| |
| |
| |
| |
| ADDL: |

Visit www.Joyefit.com for printable PDF version of **The Joyefit Fusion™ 21 Day Challenge**

Visit www.Joyefit.com for printable PDF version of
*The Joyefit Fusion Twenty-One-Day Challenge*

# Bibliography

Professor Sam Wang, Ph.D., *The Neuroscience of Everyday life.* Topic-Science and Mathematics, (lectures 1-36). The Teaching Company. www.thegreatcourses.com. 2010

Professor Peter Satterfield, Ph.D., *Mind-Body Medicine: The New Science of optimal health.* Topic Better Living. (lectures 1-36). The Teaching Company. www.thegreatcourses.com. 2013

Professor Richard Restak, M.D., *Optimizing Brain Fitness.* Topic Health and Wellness. (lectures 1-12). The Teaching Company. www.thegreatcourses.com 2012

Eckart Tolle. *A New Earth – Awakening to your life's purpose.* Eckart Tolle. A Plume Book. www.penguin,com 2005

*Merriam Webster's collegiate Dictionary.* Tenth Edition. An Encyclopedia Britannica Company. 2000

James Gavin, Ph.D., *Lifestyle Fitness Coaching.* Human Kinetics. www.humankinetics.com. 2005

Richard Restak M.D., *The Brain has a Mind of its own –insights from a practicing neurologist.* Harmony Books / New York. 1991

Frank H. Netter M.D., Sharon Colacino, Ph.D., Consulting Editor. *Atlas of Human Anatomy.* CIBA-GEIGY Corporation, pharmaceutical division. 1989

Winifred Gallagher. *The Power of Place, How Our Surroundings Shape Our Thoughts, Emotions, and Actions.* First HarperPerennial

Edition. Harper Collins Publisher, Inc. 1994

Daniel Coleman. *Working with Emotional Intelligence.* A Bantam Book. Bantam Books 1998

Daniel Kahneman. *Thinking, Fast And Slow.* Farrar, Straus and Giroux / New York. First Edition. www.fsgbooks.com. 2011

Richard Hittleman. *Richard Hittleman's Yoga 28 Day Exercise Plan.* A Bantam Book / Published by arrangement with Workman Publishing Co., Inc. Workmans Publishing Co., Inc. 1969

Robert Haas, Recipes by Hilarie Porter. *Eat Smart, Think Smart – How to use nutrients and supplements to achieve mental and physical performance.* Think Tank International Corporation. HarperCollins Publishers, Inc. 1994

Florence Scoval Shinn. *The Game of Life and How to Play it.* The Penguin Group. 1925

Rhonda Byrne. *The Power.* Atria Books. A Division of Simon and Schuster, Inc. 2010

Edward M. Hallowell, M.D., and John J. Ratey, M.D., *Driven to Distraction – Recognizing and Coping with Attention Deficit Disorder from childhood through adulthood.* First Touchstone Edition. Pantheon Books, a division of Random House, Inc. 1995

Todd Hagopian/ Hagopian Institute LLC. *Quote Junkie: Enormous Quote Book.* 2009

Daniel H. Pink. *Drive – The Surprising Truth About What Motivates Us.* Riverhead Books. The Penguin Group. 2009

Rhonda Byrne. The Secret. Atria Books. Beyond Words Publishing 2006

# Glossary

Acetylcholine: A neurotransmitter whose functions include release from the ends of the final neurons in the parasympathetic nervous system.

Adrenal glands: Glands located above the kidneys; under stress, they release catecholamine and cortisol.

Amino acids: The building blocks of proteins; about twenty different kinds, akin to letters, exist. Unique sequences of amino acids are strung together to form a particular protein. That sequence determines the folded shape of that protein and, thus, its functions.

Amygdala: An almond-shaped nucleus beneath the rostral pole of the temporal lobe; involved in the processing of emotions, particularly fear and pain, in real time and psychological pain and fear.

Androgens: A class of steroid hormones, including testosterone, with roles in aggression and sexual behavior in both sexes, but most notably in males.

Antioxidant: Antioxidants help neutralize the chemicals that cause the formation of free radicals. They are natural or synthetic chemicals or nutrients that inactivate the damaging portion of free radicals. By neutralizing free radicals, antioxidants prevent damage to cell membranes and genetic material, such as DNA.

Autonomic nervous system (ANS): A series of neural pathways originating in the hypothalamus, hindbrain, and brain stem, and projecting throughout the body; it regulates all sorts of non-conscious, automatic physiological changes throughout the body. The ANS consists of the sympathetic and parasympathetic nervous system.

Adenosine triphosphate (ATP): The universal energy molecule in nature. ATP is created in the mitochondria (energy center of each cell) by using the energy derived from foods that we consume. ATP is split by enzymes, creating the energy released for muscular contractions and various cellular functions.

Axon: The process of a neuron specialized for the transmission of information; axons are the physical structures that connect different areas of the brain.

Basal ganglia: A number of nuclei located subcortically in the forebrain. Many of the basal ganglia nuclei are involved in the extrapyramidal motor system.

Brain_stem: the part of the brain consisting of the midbrain, met encephalon, and mesencephalon.

Catecholamine: A group of brain neurotransmitters (chemicals that communicate messages between nerves), including norepinephrine and dopamine. All catecholamine's are synthesized from the amino acids L-phenylalanine and L-tyrosine.

Central nervous system (CNS): The part of the nervous system comprising the brain and the spinal cord.

Cerebellum: Part of the mesencephalon; involved in motor coordination and some cognitive functions.

Cholesterol: Manufactured in the liver and other cells. Cholesterol is found in animal protein, fats, oils, some shellfish, and egg yolks. The body uses cholesterol to synthesize hormones and cell membranes. High levels of the cholesterol known as low-density lipids (LDL) are associated with increased risk of cardiovascular disease and suspected in damaging arteries.

Cerebral cortex: The outer sheet or mantle of cells covering the hemispheres of the brain.

Chromium: An element required for the metabolism of carbohydrates. Chromium helps insulin clear the blood of glucose and move it into the cells.

Cognitive/cognition: Related to mental activities, such as thinking, learning, and memory.

Consciousness: The awareness of oneself and the world in a subjective sense.

Cortisol: A hormone produced by the adrenal cortex in response to stress. Cortisol's primary function is to increase blood sugar levels as it aids in carbohydrate and fat metabolism. Cortisol plays an important role in the stress response, cardiovascular health, and immune system.

Corpus callosum: A bundle of nerve fibers that connects the two hemispheres of the brain.

Dementia: A progressive mental deterioration.

Dendrite: The part of the neuron that receives signals from other neurons. Dendrites tend to come in the form of highly branched cables coming from the cell body of a neuron.

Depression: A disorder of mood characterized by an internal subjective state of hopelessness and despair. Depression can be brought on by a situation that creates an imbalance in brain chemistry. In these circumstances, it can be cured by balancing the brain's chemistry.

Dimethylaminothanol (DMAE): A nutrient that provides the raw materials for the synthesis of choline and acetylcholine.

DNA: The genetic blueprint that resides in the nucleus of every cell in every living organism.

Dopamine: A neurotransmitter whose functions include a role in sequential thought, the anticipation of pleasure, and aspects of fine motor control. Dopamine is also the main reward neurotransmitter and plays a major role in immune function, motivation, physical energy, and insulin regulation. Dopamine is required for short-term memory and maintaining balance in the central nervous system.

Emotion: A basic, physiological state characterized by identifiable autonomic or bodily changes.

Endorphin: Any of a group of proteins with potent analgesic properties that occur naturally in the brain. Endorphins are essentially the body's natural pain reliever.

Enzymes: Complex proteins that are capable of inducing chemical changes in other substances without being changed themselves.

Epinephrine (a.k.a. adrenaline): Both a neurotransmitter throughout the brain and a hormone released in the adrenal gland during stress as a result of activation of the sympathetic nervous system.

Fats: Fatty acids are the molecular components of fats and oils. They come in several categories: saturated, monounsaturated, and polyunsaturated.

Frontal cortex: A recently evolved region of the brain that plays a central role in executive cognitive function, decision making, gratification postponement, and regulation of the limbic system.

Free radical: A highly chemically reactive atom, molecule, or molecular fragment with a free or unpaired electron. Free radicals have been implicated in aging, cancer, cardiovascular disease, and other kinds of damage to the body. Free radicals are chaotic, imbalanced cells that damage healthy cells, rendering them unhealthy.

Gamma-aminobutyric acid (GABA): A major inhibitory neurotransmitter of the central nervous system, particularly of interneurons. For example, GABA is necessary to restore the brain's balance after a fight-or-flight episode.

Ginkgo biloba: An herbal extract from the ginkgo tree that, when dosed properly, stimulates cerebral circulation and improves mental functioning.

Glutamate: Glutamate is an excitatory neurotransmitter with critical roles in learning and memory.

Gray matter: Areas where there are collections of neuronal cell bodies.

Growth hormones: A hormone secreted by the pituitary gland that stimulates growth and repair of the body, as well as the immune system. The release of HGH is diminished with age.

Hippocampus: The hippocampus is a brain region within the limbic system that plays a central role in learning and memory.

Homeostasis: Balance, as used here. For example, balance between the sympathetic and parasympathetic portions of the autonomic nervous system. In regards to the brain's chemistry, homeostasis works on the balance between dopamine and serotonin.

Hormones: Blood-borne chemical messengers between cells, such as growth hormones, testosterone, or insulin.

Hypothalamus: A limbic structure that receives heavy input from other parts of the limbic system; plays a central role in regulating both the autonomic nervous system and hormone release.

Inhibitory neurotransmitter: A neurotransmitter that decreases the electrochemical activity of neurons. GABA and serotonin are inhibitory neurotransmitters.

Inositol: A sugar-related smart nutrient that promotes sleep when used with vitamin B3 (niacinamide) and GABA.

Law of Attraction (quantum mechanics): In physics, the law of attraction is the electric or magnetic force that acts between oppositely charged bodies, tending to draw them together. To attract by some mysterious way people, things, circumstances, and situations that appeal in either a negative or positive way that corresponds to our emotions or energy. Like energy attracts like energy.

L-arginine: An amino acid that stimulates the release of two growth hormones: insulin and human growth hormone. L-arginine is used by the body to assist in the disposal of ammonia that accumulates during protein metabolism.

L-carnitine: A molecule synthesized in the body that moves fatty acids in and out of the mitochondria, where it is burned for energy. It also stimulates the synthesis of the universal energy molecule, adenosine triphosphate (ATP).

L-taurine: An amino acid that helps protect the eye from free-radical damage and acts as a regulatory and inhibitory neurotransmitter in the brain.

L-tryptophan: An amino acid used in the synthesis of serotonin that also helps relieve pain and produces a relaxed, sleepy state when consumed with carbohydrate-rich foods.

L-tyrosine: An amino acid that is a precursor of dopamine and norepinephrine, found in high concentrations in the brain.

L-phenylalanine: An amino acid that is a precursor for the neurotransmitter norepinephrine

Limbic system: A part of the brain most strikingly involved in emotion. Some major parts include the hippocampus, amygdala, hypothalamus, and septum.

Neuron: Specialized cells of the nervous system; the structural and functional unit of the nervous system.

Nerve: A cell that carries information to and from the central nervous system.

Neurotransmitter: Small molecules used by the brain to transmit signals across synapse from one neuron to another; carries impulses between nerve cells.

Norepinephrine (a.k.a. noradrenaline): An excitatory neurotransmitter involved in alertness, concentration, aggression, and motivation. It is made in the brain from the amino acids L-phenylalnine and L-tyrosine

Opioids: Naturally occurring morphine like peptides in the brain.

Orbitofrontal cortex: A part of the frontal lobe involved in impulse control, inculcation of mores, and ability to appreciate the consequences of one's behavior.

Oxytocin: The love molecule; a peptide hormone released by the hypothalamus; plays a role in a number of processes, including bonding in social animals and humans. Oxytocin is released during childbirth and with the feelings of love, compassion, caring, sharing, bonding, trust, touch, forgiveness, empathy, and doing good for others.

Parietal lobe: A cortical lobe bordered by the central sulcus of Rolando anteriorly, the parieto-occipital sulcus posteriorly, and the Sylvian (lateral) fissure inferiorly.

Parkinson's disease: A neurodegenerative disease resulting from the loss of neurons in the substantia nigria of the midbrain; characterized by a resting tremor, abnormal posture, and paucity of normal movement.

Parasympathetic nervous system: Part of the peripheral autonomic nervous system associated with rest and digestion functions.

Parietal lobe: A cortical lobe bordered by the central suleus of Rolando anteriorly, the parieto-occipital sulcus posteriorly, and the Sylvian (lateral) fissure inferiorly.

Perception: The mental process or act of awareness on an object or idea.

Pituitary gland: A gland at the base of the brain that secretes several different hormones involved in key metabolic processes. One of the major hormones stimulated by the PG is human growth hormone (HGH).

Post-traumatic stress disorder (PTSD): A disorder characterized by anxiety and fear acquired because of a traumatic event.

Prefrontal cortex: Part of the frontal lobe implicated in working memory.

Protein: One of five categories of organic molecules present in all organisms. A protein consists of a chain of amino acids, the sequence of which is determined by information encoded in the genome. Proteins can act as enzymes and/or as structural components of organisms.

Placebo: An inert compound given to a portion of the subjects in a scientific experiment to distinguish the psychological effects from the experiment from the psychological effects of the drug being used.

Potassium: A mineral responsible for transmitting electrical impulses. It is highly active in brain tissue and the nervous system.

Precursor: A chemical that can be converted by the body into another.

Receptors: Sites on the outside of cells where particular messenger molecules, such as hormones, can attach. This attachment to the receptor site causes corresponding changes within the cell.

Ribonucleic acid (RNA): A nucleic acid that controls the protein synthesis in all cells. RNA is required for memory. Animal studies suggest that supplementing RNA may improve memory.

Serotonin: An inhibitory neurotransmitter required for sleep, relaxation, satisfaction, and stress-reduction. Serotonin helps balance the stress hormones stimulated by the fight-or-flight response.

Stroke: A rupture in a blood vessel in the brain, often with disastrous effects, depending on where the rupture occurs. The lack of blood flow or bleeding into the brain determines the damage.

Synapse: The gap between nerve cells (neurons). Chemicals called neurotransmitters are the substance that allows nerves to communicate with each other across the synaptic gaps.

Synergy: The actions of two or more compounds combined such that their effects are greater than the sum of their individual effects. For example, the nutrient OPCs is an antioxidant similar to vitamins C and E, but in addition to its own antioxidant properties, it also influences the body to recycle C and E, thereby causing the synergistic effect.

www.ingramcontent.com/pod-product-compliance
Lightning Source LLC
Chambersburg PA
CBHW030252290526
45785CB00001B/53